BUS

D1118098

How to
Save on

PRESCRIPTION
DRUGS

20 COST-SAVING METHODS

by Edward Jardini, MD

CELESTIAL ARTS
Berkeley | Toronto

The information contained in this book is based on the experience and research of the
author. It is not intended as a substitute for consulting with your physician or other
health-care provider. Any attempt to diagnose and treat an illness should be done under
the direction of a health-care professional. The publisher and author are not responsible
for any adverse effects or consequences resulting from the use of any of the suggestions,
preparations, or procedures discussed in this book.

Many of the designations used by manufacturers and sellers to distinguish their products
are claimed as trademarks. Where the publisher is aware of a trademark claim, such designations, in this book, have initial capital letters.

Celestial Arts
an imprint of Ten Speed Press
PO Box 7123
Berkeley, California 94707
www.tenspeed.com

Distributed in Australia by Simon and Schuster Australia, in Canada by Ten Speed Press
Canada, in New Zealand by Southern Publishers Group, in South Africa by Real Books,
and in the United Kingdom and Europe by Publishers Group UK.

Cover and text design by Toni Tajima

Library of Congress Cataloging-in-Publication Data
Jardini, Edward.
How to save on prescription drugs : 20 cost-saving methods / by Edward Jardini.
          p. cm.
Includes index.
Summary: "Twenty physician-recommended ways to save thousands of dollars per year on
prescription drugs"—Provided by publisher.
ISBN 978-1-58761-331-9
1. Drugs—Costs. 2. Drugs—Prices. 3. Consumer education. I. Title.

RS100.J37 2008
615'.1—dc22

                    2008004489

Printed in the United States of America on recycled paper (15% PCW)
First printing 2008

1 2 3 4 5 6 7 8 9 10 — 12 11 10 09 08

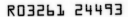
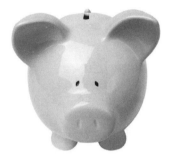

This book is dedicated to renewing faith in the art of medicine, where curing disease and maintaining health are the rewards above all others.

Contents

Acknowledgments

I WOULD LIKE TO THANK THE FOLLOWING PEOPLE for their constant encouragement to me in undertaking and completing this project: Dr. Steven Mulder, Lori Peelen, Mary La Porte, Susan Swift, Fr. Kenneth Beason, and to everyone at the Cambria Writers' Group, especially Juddi Morris. Without your belief in me, this book could never have been written.

Many thanks also to those who plodded through the early drafts: Dr. Mark Sada, Dennis Baeyen, Margaret Bayer, Dr. Cynthia Douglas, Laura Wheeler, Martha Wilson, Terry Proud, Christine Balogh, Dr. Todd Lomelino, Pamela Smith, Dr. Steven Douglass, and Cathy Stapleton. Your feedback was essential in shaping and refining the book.

Thank you to Diane Draze, Steve Wheeler, Gwen Freeman, and Andre Jardini for adept business, technical, and legal advice (often at odd hours). I am forever indebted.

Special recognition goes to Jo Ann Deck at Celestial Arts, who believed in this book when others did not, and to my editor, Lisa Westmoreland, whose expert and patient guidance tamed my wild prose into a cohesive manuscript.

Finally, immeasurable gratitude goes to my wife, Pamela (my in-house editor), and children, Elaina and Mathew, whose love and devotion sustain me, and without whom such accomplishments would have no meaning.

Introduction

"Doc, every time I go to the drugstore, I feel like I got a gun in my back. Prescription costs are robbing all of my savings!"

Mr. Merton was a retired service-station owner. He had saved diligently for his golden years, amassing what should have been an adequate nest egg. He had Medicare and a good supplemental insurance plan. His hospitalization a year and a half earlier and the placement of two coronary artery stents had been completely covered by insurance. But his medications were not a covered benefit, and they were costing him $680 per month! He calculated that at the present rate he would deplete his retirement savings in six years.

I looked over Mr. Merton's drug list. The prescribing, mostly by his cardiologist, was impeccable. Only one problem—the patient was drowning in pharmacy bills.

After an examination, we explored ways to make his treatment more affordable. We discovered that he had completed the usual course of one expensive drug that could now be stopped. Two medications were from classes that had cheaper generic members that could be substituted, and we found that another was available in a higher-strength tablet that could be split. Then I called his cardiologist. Not only was the specialist sensitive to our patient's plight, but he encouraged us to go ahead with the treatment changes.

Pleased with the prospects, Mr. Merton left the office with the new prescriptions. He returned weeks later, again feeling well. His blood pressure was excellent, cholesterol superb, and there were no side effects. He had even seen his cardiologist, who was fully satisfied with the treatment. Then came the shocker:

"The new prescriptions only cost me $84 a month."

Amazing, $600 in savings for a month of medication! How could this be? Simply by making careful medication choices, this man could now afford to continue the treatment he needed.* From then on, I paid closer attention to how prescribing practices could maintain the same high standard but also save patients money. I realized that it is not a coincidence that we physicians prescribe expensive drugs—it is not just tough luck if your doctor chooses costly medicines for you. The system is designed this way.

You see, doctors are seduced into expensive prescribing habits by a multibillion-dollar drug industry intent on maximizing profits. A barrage of promotions arrives daily in our offices. Medical journals packed with glossy drug advertisements stack up on our nightstands. We are invited to sponsored lectures, posh dinner meetings, and paid teleconferences, all pushing expensive drugs. Sales representatives bearing gifts and catering lavish luncheons constantly entice us. They fill our offices with bright sample boxes of the latest pharmaceutical offerings—usually good products, but always patented and always expensive. If these work well enough, we soon forget

---

* Mr. Merton's medication changes with direct price comparisons are provided in detail on the *How to Save on Prescription Drugs* website, www.howtosaveondrugs.com.

previous years' remedies, and we may not bother to become acquainted with less costly ones.

With a little analysis it became shamefully obvious that—with the generous assistance of the pharmaceutical companies—our prescribing practices had become exorbitant. We were accommodating the steady depletion of our patients' savings. We were helping to hold that gun in Mr. Merton's back! But it doesn't have to be that way. Excellent and up-to-date treatment can be provided substantially cheaper if doctors and patients make it a priority. But to make it happen, patients need knowledge, and they need a plan of action.

Take Control of Prescription Costs

What if you asked your doctor, "Is there a reason you are choosing that particular cholesterol-lowering pill? Is there a cheaper equivalent that would be appropriate for me?" Those questions could save you 58 percent on a new prescription.* Calling around for the best local price, using a mail-order pharmacy, or buying via the Internet can save another 50 percent. **

Better yet, challenge the recommendation with, "I understand that my total cholesterol is 295, doctor, but since my ten-year risk assessment for cardiovascular disease is less than 1 percent, I do not need to take a cholesterol-lowering drug."

---

 * The average retail price for ninety 10 mg generic lovastatin tablets is $126, versus $298 for ninety 10 mg Lipitor.
** Drugstore.com sells 10 mg lovastatin tablets in quantity at 56 percent less than the average retail price.

This bit of knowledge saves you 100 percent of the prescription cost! *

Wouldn't you just love to challenge your doctor with questions like, "Why start treating my high blood pressure with an ARB? Wouldn't it be cheaper to try a diuretic first?" There may be a good reason for starting with an expensive ARB (over twenty times more expensive!), and your doctor will explain this. But if there isn't a good reason, you might be very well treated with the diuretic. This kind of constructive discourse can steer treatment choices toward the best option. And you don't need a medical degree to start the conversation. With the information in this book, you will be able to enlist your doctor's help in obtaining the best possible health care at an affordable price.

It was from the true story of Mr. Merton that this book emerged. I took the basic principles of that triumph and expanded upon them, drawing on the experience of more than seventy-five thousand outpatient visits logged over a twenty-year medical practice. I interviewed pharmacists, colleagues, and allied health professionals; I studied prescription drug costs, patent laws, and structuring of insurance formularies. I also researched government health care agencies and patient assistance programs. Ultimately, I developed a program of cost-saving methods that patients can use to bring prescription

---

* According to the National Cholesterol Education Program website risk calculator, a forty-year-old nonsmoking female with average systolic blood pressure of 110 and total and HDL cholesterol of 295 and 72, respectively, has a ten-year cardiovascular disease risk of less than 1 percent.

drug costs within their budgets. Over the ensuing months, I began to apply these principles to my own patients, acquiring feedback and refining the concepts further. The program worked! My patients reported affordable prescription costs, some saving hundreds of dollars each month. Close follow-up showed no compromise in medical management, and in many cases, response to treatment improved.

Who's It For?

This book was conceived for patients on long-term treatment with prescription medicines who would like to save money. Patients with chronic medical conditions treated with expensive drugs are ideally suited. Those without prescription drug coverage will certainly benefit, but even those with Medicare Part D or other prescription benefit programs will save money by using my cost-saving program. Out-of-pocket costs with any prescription drug plan will be cheaper when the total prescription burden is less. This particularly applies for Medicare patients whose prescription costs put them into the "doughnut hole" or coverage gap. However, almost anyone taking prescription drugs can benefit.

How Does It Work?

The cost-saving methods are described briefly chapter by chapter with only enough patient sketches and examples to quickly illustrate the concepts. Some methods are merely clever tricks (such as splitting higher-dose tablets) that require only a few pages of explanation but can cut medication costs significantly, once you know how. Some of the cost-saving methods show you how to dodge expensive industry traps or even treat your medical condition effectively without prescription drugs. Still others deal with obtaining prescription medicines at the best possible price or even free. Information on qualifying for assistance and government programs is also given. I have even added a chapter on the new Medicare prescription drug plans, explaining how to use them to your best advantage.

Most of the methods require the support of your doctor. Your doctor must become a partner for affordable health care. This alliance is made at a specialized office visit I call the "treatment review visit." This encounter will be different from a typical office visit, so directions on how to prepare, schedule, and conduct the visit are given in detail.

The end of the book features the Expensive-Drug Survival Index, which lists cheaper alternatives to popular costly drugs that you can discuss with your doctor. Case studies in the chapters show examples of how the methods were used to help real patients. It is compelling to see how careful medication choices and other strategies can lower treatment costs and improve medical care. Some of the strategies will correlate to your own treatments, and inspire money-saving ideas to present at your treatment review.

Additional Benefits

This book is not only about saving money. It should also stimulate improved communication and cooperation between doctor and patient. I can speak from experience that knowledgeable, interactive patients get more attention and diligence from their physicians. This, in turn, fosters better patient compliance and better response to treatment. It promotes a satisfying synergy between doctor and patient. By enlisting your doctor in a program to treat you effectively and *affordably*, both of you should feel a renewed enthusiasm and sense of partnership for good health.

Unfortunately, commercialism in the pharmaceutical industry has misdirected the primary goal of medical therapy from promoting health to promoting profits. My program challenges that trend. In the explanations of the cost-saving methods, many profiteering schemes are exposed. As patients begin to schedule treatment review visits and discuss cost-saving methods, doctors will see how their prescribing practices have been manipulated to maximize company profits. Once enlightened about industry craftiness, physicians can return to a refined, evidence-based approach to medical treatment. Thus, this book may become a small part of a health care revolution that needs to take place in the United States, resulting in freedom from commercial interference. But it will only start when patients enlist physician support and refuse to be denied affordable care.

Regarding Drug Prices and Patient Names

All prices of drugs in the text are the average retail price for a ninety-day supply at the usual lowest starting dose as listed on Drugstore.com as of March 2008 unless otherwise indicated. (Average retail price is the discount Internet price plus the savings given in parethesis.) All of the prices listed in certain clearly-marked drug tables are the discount retail prices from the same source and date and are indicated as the "discount Internet price." These were chosen because the average retail price may not have been available for all of the drugs in that table, and to keep direct price comparisons valid. Discount Internet prices will probably be lower than those at most retail outlets. Prescription drug prices fluctuate, so the prices given in this book should be considered estimates and not necessarily the current rate. Actual prices may vary. For clarification, brand-name drugs appear capitalized; generic drugs are lowercased.

Patient names have been changed to preserve anonymity and confidentiality.

Final Note

Finally, let me state that I am in no way affiliated or directly financially involved with any drug manufacturer, retailer, or any other commercial interest mentioned in this book. The names of the specific businesses and services cited are given only as a possible means of assistance to the reader in obtaining prescription medications at an affordable price.

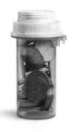

1

The Treatment Review Visit

"WHY CAN'T YOU DOCTORS PRESCRIBE drugs your patients can afford?"

The question did not come from a patient, but rather from a pharmacist friend who works at our local Wal-Mart. He was talking about how his customers react when confronted with the cost of prescriptions. "I've seen people take items out of the basket so they'll have enough to cover their medicines," he went on. "Sometimes they ask me, 'Which ones should I get?' because they can't afford to buy them all."

A patient of mine summarized the reality of prescription drug purchases for many when she stated plainly, "I buy what I can afford to pay for." The problem is not uncommon. In a nationwide survey of more than four thousand patients over age fifty, 18 percent reported taking less than their prescribed dose of medication due to cost. Twenty-two percent cut back on essentials, including food, to pay for prescription drugs. Amazingly, 84 percent of these patients had some type of prescription benefit plan! Even more disturbing were the results that only 16 percent reported being asked by a doctor or nurse whether they could afford their medications.[1] These statistics reflect the sorry state of affordability of medications for many people in this country. Worse, they show just how unaware American physicians are about their patients' ability to pay for the drugs they prescribe.

Doctors are expected to keep up with medical advances. Our licenses and specialty status depend on completion of a certain amount of continuing medical education. This is the way we keep current on the latest, most effective treatments including the "drugs of choice" for each disease. But rarely is there any discussion of the financial burden to patients. There seems to be an underlying notion among the medical community that somehow all of the marvelous new treatments will be available to everyone.

In a January 2006 letter to the *Los Angeles Times*, Dr. Larry S. Fields, president of the American Academy of Family Practice, wrote, "In my practice I treat many seniors with chronic conditions requiring medication, often expensive medication. Some of my patients have tapped their savings to cover the cost of medication. Others have gone without, with serious implications."[2] This admission by a notable physician was offered as testament to the validity of the new Medicare prescription drug program, but it caused me to wonder, "Why was Dr. Fields prescribing medicines that his patients could not afford? Was he unaware of the discrepancy between their means and the cost of treatment?"

A young woman with insulin-dependent diabetes returned to a family practice colleague after consultation with a specialist. The patient was in tears. She told my colleague that the specialist had outlined a treatment plan that the young woman couldn't possibly afford. And she had health insurance! What good was the specialist's expertise if the patient received no benefit? Yet he probably completed his day feeling satisfied that he had given the most up-to-date treatment advice to each of his patients. Why didn't he know this patient might not be able to afford it? Well, for one thing, she didn't tell him.

Who will reveal the truth to doctors about prescription costs? Who is going to teach us to consider patient means when prescribing drug therapy? It certainly won't be our medical journals, which are almost entirely sponsored by the drug companies; leaf through the first twenty pages of any copy of the *New England Journal of Medicine* and you will see page after page of advertising for expensive prescription drugs. It isn't going to be the AMA; they are more concerned with *doctors'* financial health than patients'. It's not going to be the Surgeon General or the Department of Health and Human Services, nor will it be the university medical centers or the National Institutes of Health. They've all had their chances, and look where we are today: one of five elderly Americans choosing between food and medicine. Who, then?

You.

Patients like you are going to do it. Visit by visit, one doctor at a time, patients are going to bring the message that drug treatment must be tailored to their ability to afford it. Remember that medicine is a service industry and that your doctor works for you. Directly or indirectly, your doctor is paid for the service he provides to you. Wouldn't you tell a hired serviceman if he was not doing a good job? If you cannot pay for the treatment your doctor recommends or have to sacrifice essentials to get it, you are not getting your money's worth at the office visit; he is not giving you good service.

It is certainly not my intention to create animosity between you and your doctor—quite the opposite. I am trying to break through traditional barriers that might prevent you from obtaining reasonably priced medical care. People are usually quite respectful of physicians, particularly at their appointments. The doctor is a knowledgeable, authoritative figure. How could you possibly question his recommendations? The answer is simple: just remember *he* works for *you*. Instead of crying to her family doctor, the young diabetic woman should have informed the specialist as soon as she realized she could not afford his treatment plan. Dr. Fields' patients likewise should have protested his medication choices. Most patients have never confronted a doctor in that way. Many would be embarrassed or afraid to do so. But this chapter will show you how to approach your doctor—your service provider—in order to obtain affordable treatment.

Train Your Doctor to Work for You

To economize treatment, you need to form a partnership with your doctor—a collaboration that strives for the best possible health care at a reasonable price. This alliance might be initiated at any office appointment, but I recommend a dedicated consultation I call the treatment review visit. Let's face it; the doctor's day is unpredictable and disrupted by urgent situations and unexpected emergencies. This is partly why you languish so long in the waiting room. If you try to add a discussion of medication costs to your usual visit, you may be slighted. There just isn't enough time for the doctor to make an assessment of ongoing problems, perform an examination, evaluate and treat new concerns, and also make a meaningful appraisal of treatment costs. A comprehensive review of medications is fundamental and should not be rushed. If it enables you to afford treatment, it is worth a dedicated visit, and you will need to make a specific appointment to start the process.

Get Ready to Save

Schedule an appointment with your doctor to review your medications. Don't attempt to initiate treatment changes with phone calls, faxes, letters, or emails. Treatment changes are too elaborate for those forms of communication. Fostering an affordable health alliance requires an intimate dialogue that only a face-to-face office visit can provide. Insist the visit be with your usual doctor, not a partner or associate, nurse, or physician's assistant. Request an adequate amount of time for the visit, at least thirty minutes for every two or three expensive drugs you take. Make the receptionist aware that the purpose of the appointment will be only to review treatment and medication costs.

Before the visit, you must prepare. Like an attorney giving arguments at trial, you will make your case for affordable treatment, and you must be ready. First, add up your current prescription costs. Then determine a medication budget (see chapter 2), and be ready to show the shortfall. Next, prepare suggestions for changes to the treatment plan with the projected savings. These are explained in the cost-saving methods and case studies in the following chapters.

Conducting a Treatment Review Visit

When the doctor arrives, quickly let her know that you do not want an examination but are only there to discuss your medications. Impress upon her your present medication costs and what your budget will allow. Tell her you appreciate that each medication has been carefully chosen, but make it clear that the present regimen is not acceptable.

"I need your help, doctor," is a great way to start. "I cannot afford the drugs you prescribe."

If it's true, admit that you've skipped or reduced doses or have gone without essentials due to the cost.

"I never filled the prescription for Advair because it costs over $200 a month!"

This statement emphasizes the urgency and gives grounds that something must change. Don't let her off the hook if she offers free drug samples! Counter with *this*:

"Unless you can guarantee a lifetime supply, those samples won't solve my problem."

Then tell her you'd like to streamline treatment by eliminating medicines that are no longer necessary:

"Doc, we keep adding new drugs for blood pressure, diabetes, and cholesterol, but we never get rid of any. Is every drug I take necessary?"

Anyone taking four or more medicines should definitely start with a similar question. This forces your doctor to focus on management of complicated long-term medical problems, considering the value of each drug at the present point in time. Hopefully, therapies that are no longer beneficial are recognized and eliminated. Start the analysis with questions such as, "The test showed that my duodenal ulcer was healed a year ago. Is there any reason to continue the Nexium?" or, "It's been more than a year since I felt depressed. Shall we try weaning me off Cymbalta now?" You can also request confirmation of a diagnosis or that a particular drug was ever necessary. Don't be shy; it's your health and your money.

"My previous doctor started me on Singulair. It's quite expensive, and I'm not sure why I take it. Is it really necessary?"

This statement would have served Greta Barker well. She was a new patient taking Singulair along with thirteen other prescription drugs. Singulair is a costly second-line therapy for resistant cases of asthma and allergies, but Greta had neither condition. Records showed that a hospital doctor started the drug while she was under treatment for pneumonia. She was sent home with a prescription her family doctor continued to refill, costing her $338 every three months. With supervision, Greta stopped taking Singulair without any ill effect to her health but with substantial benefit to her bank account! (Cost-saving method 4.)

You *could* just say your medications are too expensive and ask about alternatives. However, you are more likely to engage the physician if you offer specific proposals. This is also your opportunity to begin your doctor's education in economical prescribing! Single out an expensive medication and show her a cost-saving method:

- "The 10 mg Lexapro tablets cost $300 for ninety tablets. Splitting a 20 mg tablet cuts the cost in half and saves me $600 a year!" (Cost-saving method 13.)

- "Generic metoprolol twice a day instead of brand-name Toprol-XL is one-tenth the cost! Switching to the generic would save me over $350 a year." (Cost-saving method 10.)

- "The Norvasc controls my blood pressure, but $220 for a three month supply is outrageous. I understand a diuretic can work as well or better at just pennies per pill." (Cost-saving method 12.)

- "The neurologist prescribes me three 100 mg Neurontin capsules to take at a time. A single 300 mg capsule provides the same dose of the same drug and saves $415 a year!" (Cost-saving method 14.)

- "Could we try changing my cholesterol drug from Lipitor to generic lovastatin? That would save me over $1,000 a year." (Cost-saving method 11.)

- "I understand that treatment of women with a bone density T-score above −2.5 with Fosamax has shown little to no benefit in prevention of fractures. I'd rather save the $1,200 a year and continue with nonprescription prevention." (Cost-saving method 7.)

These proposals may sound too sophisticated for you to make, but believe me, they are not. The chapters that follow will show you how to do it. You only need to know how the cost-saving methods apply to *your* treatment, not to every medical therapy.

Your doctor may approve a proposed treatment change or suggest an alternative plan. Keep an open mind and respect her counsel. Some of your ideas may not be suited to your particular case. Your doctor needs your input on medication costs, but you need her expertise in medical management. It is also wise not to make too many changes at once; one at a time is best. That way, if you experience an adverse effect, you can deduce what change in therapy caused it.

By the end of the initial treatment review visit, you will have delivered a powerful message. I guarantee your doctor will not forget this encounter. From that day forward she will respect your need for economy in prescribing and begin to treat more reasonably with drugs.

Follow-Up

When changes are made, request timely follow-up to assess results and make adjustments. If a change of therapy doesn't work out, perhaps due to an adverse reaction, do not be discouraged. And don't be too anxious to go back to the original treatment, the one you couldn't afford. Remember that prohibitive cost is an intolerable side effect too. There are usually multiple alternatives to treatment with an expensive drug. If a cheaper medication causes side effects, try the next option. Eventually you will arrive at a well-tolerated, effective, *and affordable* treatment.

> Within three months, Greta Barker's drug costs were brought under control. Her medication list was reduced from 14 to 7 drugs, and her monthly pharmacy bill dropped from $1,290 to $170, a savings of more than $13,000 per year.

The cost-saving methods are explained simply and thoroughly in the chapters that follow. Case studies give practical examples of affordable alternatives to the most popular, expensive drugs. As you read, jot down ideas and proposals for cutting costs that apply to your treatment. Ultimately, you will be ready to begin training your doctor to prescribe treatment that you can afford.

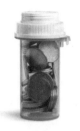

2

Budgeting Prescription Costs

Primum non nocere. (First, do no harm.)

—Hippocrates (circa 460–377 B.C.E.)

AT THE TIME YOUR DOCTOR recommends treatment with medication, it is quite likely that neither of you have any idea what it costs. Starting a patient out with a bagful of drug company samples of uncertain retail price is unconscionable. This common practice completely removes the doctor from any financial discussion. The unfortunate patient then stands alone in shock at the drugstore counter when he ultimately has to buy more pills. Where is the doctor-patient relationship at that moment of revelation? When the physician does not know how much a new treatment is going to cost, and the patient unwittingly accepts it, I call it *idiopathic prescribing*: the patient is pathetic, and the doctor is an idiot!

Your doctor may be a brilliant clinician with knowledge of the latest clinical studies and all the newest drugs. Nevertheless, if he prescribes treatment that needlessly punches a large draining hole into your savings account, you should consider a divorce. The familiar doctor's motto, "First, do no harm," should also apply to the patient's wallet. Physicians have an *obligation* to make reasonable recommendations. This includes affordable prescribing.

What's It Gonna Cost?

As a patient, you are also a consumer. You must check the price tag before heading to the checkout counter. When your doctor recommends a new therapy with a prescription drug, find out what it costs. A vague response from the physician is not adequate. If the doctor doesn't know the price, show him how to get it! Prices can be quickly found at CVS.com or another online website. Everybody has cellular telephones these days. (Many patients think nothing of taking a call during my examination!) Why not call the local drugstore before leaving the office? That will get the doctor's attention! You could get the bad news at the drug store, but if the price is unacceptably high, you are left with the hassle of calling the office, leaving a message with the staff, waiting for a return call, and so on. You know the routine. And the next prescription may be more expensive than the first! No, it is better to discuss every facet of a new treatment face to face with the doctor, including the expense. Be adamant. Tell her, "Doctor, before I can start this medication, I must know the cost." If you are already overburdened with medication costs, the methods described later in this book will help. But first you must determine a prescription budget.

How Much Have You Got?

You may have no problem with ongoing treatment with medications costing even three or four dollars per day. Lipitor, a popular drug for high cholesterol, costs about $140 for a month of treatment. But consider the drug Casodex for prostate cancer: it'll set you back $567 per month. Could you afford it? How about Enbrel, a drug for rheumatoid arthritis priced at $1,800 a month? Rebif, for multiple sclerosis, goes for $2,374. Could you afford the drug Somavert? A month of treatment is over $8,000!

Most patients will not encounter these extremes, but the examples show that almost anyone's cash pool could be severely siphoned by prescription costs. So what is your medication budget? How much can you afford to pay month in and month out for drug treatment? You can't expect your doctor to prescribe within your means if she doesn't know what you can manage. If insurance isn't picking up the entire tab, you must honestly disclose the limitations of your budget to the doctor whenever the prescription pad comes out.

There are many ways to determine a medication budget. Some people can estimate a fairly accurate monthly allowance for medical treatment without having to sharpen a pencil. Others whose means are more meager, or whose medication costs are very high, will find it necessary to do some reckoning.

Start with your monthly income. Include social security, pensions, investment and rental income, stipends, alimony, salary, and wages. What portion of savings or other principal can be drawn upon? You don't want to completely deplete your savings in your lifetime. Now subtract expenses: mortgage or rent, utilities, transportation costs, insurance, services, food, and clothing. Medications should take priority over most nonessential expenses, but how much income to delegate to items such as travel and entertainment is a personal decision. How much of the monthly income is left, and what percentage of that can you reasonably apportion for medical treatment? That is the figure you must present to your doctor.

Take It to the Bank

- Determine the monthly amount you can afford to spend on medications.
- Add up your current monthly medication costs. Are you within your budget?
- Convey these amounts to your doctor at the treatment review visit and whenever medication changes are proposed.
- Using the cost-saving methods, work with your physician to keep prescription costs within budget.
- Insist on learning the cost of proposed drug therapies when they are first prescribed. Discuss the impact of these treatments on your prescription budget with your doctor.
- Notify your doctor whenever prescription costs exceed your budget so that cheaper alternatives can be explored or discounts or assistance programs can be sought.

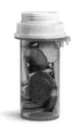

3

Eliminate Nonessential Prescriptions

Cost-Saving Methods 1 through 4

Clinicians tend to err on the side of pharmacologic solutions to any medical problem; they fail to reevaluate medication lists at every clinical encounter; and they are subject to the reflex refilling of prescriptions even after initial indications for the medication have disappeared.[1]

–Allan S. Brett, MD, editor in chief, *Journal Watch*

THE TITLE OF THIS CHAPTER might sound absurdly obvious, but I am serious. Ongoing treatment with medication that is no longer necessary, no longer effective, or has never been necessary or effective wastes more of the prescription dollar than anything else. Discontinuation of nonessential medications may not only result in significant savings but also improve your general health. Every unnecessary medication removed from your treatment eliminates a risk of adverse side effects and drug interactions. But surely every medicine your doctor's office refills month after month is absolutely necessary and effective, isn't it? Hardly.

A team of physicians and pharmacists looked at how often unnecessary drugs were prescribed to patients discharged from several US Veterans Affairs hospitals. The researchers found at least one unnecessary drug prescribed to 44 percent of the patients. Nearly one in five received *two or more* unnecessary prescriptions! Duplication of treatments and a lack of proven benefit were some of the common reasons that the drugs were judged inappropriate. In many cases no justification for a particular treatment could be found.[2]

Think that only happens at the VA? I know of a recent patient at my local community hospital who was discharged with twenty-six different prescriptions! Every one of those must have been necessary and effective, right? In 2001, the *Journal of the American Medical Association* found that 23 percent of older US adults studied received at least one drug judged inappropriate to their treatment.[3]

There are several reasons why some of your drugs could be eliminated, but let me first emphasize that you should not discontinue any medical treatment except in conjunction with your physician. This is preferably done at the treatment review visit. If the information herein and a personal review of your medications lead you to suspect that a particular treatment may not be essential, jot down your concerns and see your doctor. Continue all prescribed treatments in the meantime. Your doctor should be able to either justify the therapy or agree to a trial discontinuation. Either way, you will improve your understanding of the treatment and stimulate more effective communication with your doctor. And, you just may be taken off an unnecessary and expensive medication.

CSM 1: Eliminate Medicines That Are No Longer Needed

Sure, the Nexium relieved your heartburn last year. The upper endoscopy was normal. You've lost some weight, you've cut down on caffeine and alcohol, and you're eating better. Perhaps you don't need the drug anymore. Maybe you could take it on an as-needed basis instead of daily. Maybe an over-the-counter antacid would do as well. If it is not obvious what a medicine is doing for you now, at this point in time, ask your doctor if it might be discontinued.

Most prescription treatments are not meant to be continued indefinitely. Nevertheless, thousands of patients continue swallowing drugs month after month, year after year, to the detriment of their bank accounts and perhaps their health. It baffles me how many patients taking prescriptions repeatedly postpone—or try to avoid altogether—follow-up visits with their doctors. It's as if they have gotten away with something if they can get their medicines refilled without a doctor's visit. This attitude completely misses the point of the follow-up appointment. There should be periodic assessment of every medical problem and treatment, at which time changes in management can take place. If there is no office visit, there can be no change in therapy, and no chance to take a course of treatment to conclusion. Of course, a doctor's appointment could also result in additional prescriptions, but hopefully that would mean improved disease management and better health.

If you are under treatment with prescription medicines for high blood pressure, diabetes, or high cholesterol, and you have made the recommended lifestyle changes, chances are that some of your medicines can be reduced or eliminated. Even a modest reduction in weight enables many patients to come off of prescription drugs. I am not talking about achieving "ideal body weight." Ten or fifteen pounds of weight loss is often enough to allow a downsizing of prescriptions. Obesity specialists routinely eliminate prescription treatments for these conditions in their patients who lose weight. Lifestyle changes including an improved diet, regular exercise, and permanent weight reduction are a means to regain control of your health and rely less on prescription drugs.

Feeling Fine and Not Going to Take It Anymore

There is a standard end point to drug therapy for many conditions. For instance, studies show that most peptic ulcers heal completely with eight weeks of treatment with a proton pump inhibitor (PPI) such as Aciphex, Nexium, Prevacid, or Protonix.[4] Nevertheless, many patients continue these drugs indefinitely following diagnosis of an ulcer, at a cost of $426

(Protonix) to $557 (Prevacid) every three months. Unless other conditions (such as Barrett's esophagus or chronic gastritis) are present, PPIs can be appropriately and safely discontinued after an ulcer has healed. Stopping long-term therapy with PPIs not only saves money but also might prevent a hip fracture! A December 2006 study showed that the risk of hip fracture was up to two-and-a-half times greater in patients taking high-dose PPI therapy for more than one year.[5]

How long should you take Celexa, Cymbalta, Effexor, Lexapro, Paxil, Prozac, Wellbutrin, or Zoloft for depression? There is not a universal answer, but most episodes of depression do resolve. It is only the unique case of chronic depression that requires ongoing indefinite treatment. The American Psychiatric Association Practice Guideline recommends sixteen to twenty weeks of successful drug therapy.[6] Even Pfizer, the manufacturer of the popular antidepressant Zoloft, indicates as little as "several months" to be maintenance treatment for depression. Then why is everybody taking these drugs incessantly? Well, some patients are reluctant to stop for fear of a relapse. Others try to discontinue antidepressants (or simply forget to take them) and experience withdrawal symptoms. They then become convinced that they can't get along without the stuff. Weaned off carefully, most people can avoid withdrawals and will continue to do fine without the drugs. Nonetheless, the most common reason these drugs are continued so long is—the doctor never suggests going off of them.

But even if you successfully wean yourself off an antidepressant after an appropriate period of remission, won't the depression come back? Unfortunately, recurrence of depression is common—in one study reappearing in up to a third of elderly patients within two years, *even when continuing on antidepressant medication!*[7] So it is more important to recognize the symptoms of a recurring depression, and to receive regular follow-up care from your physician, than to stay on medication indefinitely. That way, appropriate intervention can take place promptly whether you are already taking medication or not.

Warning: *Depression is a serious and life-threatening illness that should be closely monitored by a health care professional. Do not discontinue or alter treatment with medications in any way without the careful consideration and approval of a knowledgeable physician.*

Inpatient Insanity

It is becoming increasingly common for patients' hospital care to be managed by inpatient specialists called *hospitalists.* Indeed, you may never even see your personal doctor once you are admitted to the hospital. The hospitalist and perhaps a variety of specialists will direct your care in the hospital, then send you back to your family doctor after discharge. This loss of continuity can result in poor communication among the physicians and lead to inefficient and expensive prescribing. You may get back to your doctor before the hospital records do, and it may not be clear why certain medicines were started. (And you'll be on many more drugs than before you went in!) Without a detailed hospital discharge summary directing otherwise, your doctor will likely continue new prescriptions initiated during a hospital stay.

Perhaps your blood pressure was high while awaiting an elective surgery, and an antihypertension drug was administered. Will you need to continue the medicine indefinitely? A patient admitted to the intensive care unit for any number of severe conditions may be appropriately given a PPI for ulcer prevention. But in most cases, the medication can be stopped after going home. Many are prescribed analgesics, tranquilizers, laxatives, antacids, and sleeping aids to make their inpatient stay as comfortable as possible. Will your doctor know which can be safely discontinued or just keep the pharmacist's cash register singing?

Case Study
CSM 1: Eliminate Medicines That Are No Longer Needed

Francine is a seventy-eight-year-old retired antiques dealer and breast cancer survivor who came to me in March 2006. Included among her usual medicines was Fosamax, which she had taken dutifully along with calcium and vitamin D since a low bone-mineral density was discovered seven years prior by screening DEXA scan. She had no history of fractures, but her mother had in her eighties. She was of northern European descent, had smoked until five years prior, and she weighed less than 125 pounds, so preventive treatment with medication was justified.

What Francine didn't know, however, is that long-term studies of Fosamax show that after five years, there is no further reduction in overall fractures.[8] Moreover, recent data suggest that longer-term bisphosphonate therapy might be associated with actual weakening of bone and *increased* susceptibility to fractures.[9] With this information, Francine was happy to stop the expensive therapy that was no longer needed.

Yearly Savings: $1,137

CSM 2: Eliminate Medicines That No Longer Work

Whereas in CSM 1, treatment with prescription medicine is no longer required, there is another situation where a medication, although requisite, is no longer effective. Some drugs that work well initially lose their effectiveness over time. Eventually, they may no longer contribute to the treatment and become a waste of money and a source of side effects.

Still Going?

Some medications stop working due to the progression of the disease state. Avandia, metformin, and glyburide—all common treatments for diabetes—are examples. It is not unusual for the benefits of these medications to diminish after several years. A December 2006 study showed the percentage of patients failing therapy with one of these drugs after five years to be 15 percent with Avandia, 21 percent with metformin, and 34 percent with glyburide.[10] Treatment failure is not the fault of the drug, but reflects progression of the diabetes. Thankfully, other therapies are available to rescue the patient from poor blood sugar control. But when additional treatments are being considered, it is also a time to reevaluate the medicines in use and eliminate those that are no longer effective.

Other medications are prone to a phenomenon known as *tachyphylaxis*. This implies a loss of potency over time. In other words, a 5 mg dose of a drug may work fine for a while, but eventually a 10 mg dose becomes necessary to get the same effect. This is not due to the worsening of the medical condition under treatment but rather has to do with the way the body adapts to the medication over time.

Alpha-1-blockers such as Hytrin (terazosin), Cardura (doxazosin), and Minipress (prazosin) are known to exhibit tachyphyllaxis in their effect on lowering blood pressure. The clue appears when, all other things remaining stable, blood pressure starts to climb. In some cases the dose can be increased with renewed control of blood pressure. However, this may not be an option when intolerable side effects appear, or when the maximum recommended dose is reached. In these cases, the patient should be weaned off these drugs. Alpha-1-blockers, which also include Flomax (tamsulosin) and Uraxatrol (afluzosin), are also prescribed for the treatment of urinary symptoms associated with an enlarging prostate gland. Although the effectiveness of these medicines for this purpose may also wear off, it is more likely due to ongoing prostate enlargement than tachyphyllaxis. Either way, if the drug has lost effectiveness, it should be stopped.

Feeding a Habit

In medical practice, tachyphylaxis is most commonly seen with the long-term use of narcotic pain relievers. Hydrocodone (Vicodin, Norco, Lortabs, and others) is the most prescribed medicine of the last decade in the United States.

Over ninety-two million prescriptions for hydrocodone were dispensed in 2004 alone. Oxycontin/Percocet (oxycodone), Darvocet/Darvon (propoxyphine), Ultram/Ultracet (tramadol), Duragesic (fentanyl), and codeine are other narcotics commonly prescribed for pain. The use of these medications for the treatment of chronic pain has become less controversial, but the ever-increasing dose required in order to maintain adequate analgesia continues to be a problem.

Unfortunately, many patients receiving narcotics for chronic pain continue to be hampered by pain. The treatment is initially beneficial, but it becomes less so despite higher and more frequent dosing. Eventually, the patients have two problems: the pain they started with and a new dependency on narcotics. Patients taking frightfully high doses of narcotic medications often tell me that their pain is still not controlled, but that they cannot do without the drugs. At that point it is not the chronic pain but an addiction that is being treated.

When used regularly, the minor tranquilizers and some sleeping aids are also habit forming. Examples are Xanax (alprazolam), Ativan (lorazepam), Klonapin (clonazepam), Halcion (triazolam), and Restoril (temazepam). Although used for different purposes, these drugs belong to a single class called *benzodiazepines*. Xanax and Ativan are commonly used to treat anxiety disorders. Taken on a regular basis, tolerance to these drugs develops and the patient requires higher doses to control symptoms. Ironically, once habituation occurs, a missed or reduced dose can result in rebound anxiety. One then has to wonder if it is the anxiety disorder or the withdrawal that is being treated. If alleviation of withdrawal symptoms becomes the objective of further dosing of the drug, a continuing cycle of anxiety and relief is created. This is not only counterproductive but also a waste of money.

Habituation with sleeping pills results in a similar problem. Regular dosing may become required to assist with sleep. Then if a dose is missed, a long wakeful night is inevitable, the very problem you took the stuff for in the first place. Despite FDA approval for long-term use, the newer prescription sleeping aids are also likely to be associated with development of tolerance and withdrawal symptoms.

The management of chronic pain, anxiety disorders, and insomnia is challenging for both patient and physician. However, transient relief that comes with a prescription drug habit satisfies no one (except the drug manufacturers and retailers!). The cost to the patient is much higher than the price of the tablets at the pharmacy—it includes the financial burden of lost work time, the social disruption of interpersonal relationships, and the emotional loss of self-esteem. Although few people addicted to prescription drugs would endure detoxification just to save a buck, with the support of a physician and loved ones, most should do it to beat the habit and renew their lives.

It is for these patients, whose pain, anxiety, and insomnia are really no better for all of the drugs, that I recommend a complete change of therapy. Counseling, inpatient treatment, and assistance of organizations such as Narcotics Anonymous (NA) may be required. Alternative therapies including nonaddicting medications, surgery, physical therapy, chiropractic treatments, nerve blocks, epidural steroid injections, acupuncture, and hypnosis may also be successful. Treatment at a university medical center, chronic pain clinic, psychiatry practice, or sleep disorder clinic can be sought. Here, the treatment change is not so much to save money as it is to restore the patient's dignity, productivity, and self-worth, and perhaps to save his very life.

Case Study
CSM 2: Eliminate Medicines That No Longer Work

Eugene is a sixty-three-year-old retired DMV manager with diabetes. Initially, glipizide alone was sufficient to control his blood sugars. Over the years, metformin and Avandia were added to maintain control. With each added medication, blood sugars improved, but ultimately even this triple therapy did not provide adequate diabetic control. After consultation and several visits with the diabetes educator, Eugene was started on insulin therapy. Fortunately, his blood sugars responded nicely, but the three pills he took for diabetes were a financial burden. Over several weeks we decided to wean him off and discontinue each of the three diabetes pills sequentially while monitoring blood sugars several times a day. Happily, there was no loss of blood sugar control. Only minor adjustments in insulin therapy were required, and we eliminated three medications that no longer worked.

Yearly Savings: $4,143

CSM 3: Eliminate Medicines That Have Never Worked

"Why do you take this one?" I inquired of my mother-in-law as I inspected one of a dozen prescription bottles she had dumped onto our kitchen table.

"That one? I think it's for the pain in my legs."

"Does it work?"

"Not really."

"Then why do you take it?"

"Because the doctor said so!"

But You Said I Needed This!

I am bewildered by how many patients continue to take expensive prescription medicines that don't do anything for them. The drugs are started in earnest, but somehow appropriate follow-up is missed, and the treatment continues without justification.

Neurontin (gabapentin) is an antiseizure drug that was found to be effective for the treatment of neuropathic pain (pain originating in affected nerves). The medication is a godsend for many patients with chronic pain associated with shingles, diabetes, and other disorders. The benefit to these conditions is so impressive that Neurontin is now tried for almost any type of chronic pain. Unfortunately, the wider the spectrum of painful conditions treated, the more treatment failures with Neurontin we see. Many patients started on this medicine continue to take it without realizing any benefit. And the cost can be astounding: the average retail price for a three-month supply of treatment (600 mg three times a day) is $1,016.

How can this happen? How can patients spend hundreds of dollars a month on a prescription that does them no good? Well, in some cases a trial of the medication is appropriately started by a neurologist or chronic pain specialist, who then sends the patient back to the family doctor or internist for follow-up. The dutiful doctor (and faithful patient) continue the specialist's recommendation without question. No one bothers to assess if the drug has done anything. Some pain patients are so desperate for relief that they push on, taking the drug in the hope that it may eventually help. Others are simply ever-obedient to their doctors' orders, regardless of any favorable outcome.*

Continuation of ineffective medications sometimes happens in the course of managing complicated treatment protocols. The stepwise approach to the management of hypertension previously advocated by the National Institutes of Health provides an example. According to the protocol, the first medication treatment step was to prescribe a diuretic or a beta-blocker. If this therapy was ineffective, the other medicine was then added. At the next evaluation, if the combination did not meet treatment goals, a third-line medication was added, and so on until the blood pressure was controlled. At each doctor visit along the way, an assessment was made

* In fairness to Neurontin, the medicine is not always given a fair trial. It has a very broad range of dosing, from 300 mg to 3600 mg per day, which must be adjusted to the individual. If starting doses are not helpful, the dosage should be increased at intervals.

of the patient's response to treatment and any possible side effects. But medicines that had shown absolutely no effect on lowering blood pressure were often not discontinued when the next line of therapy was added. Although this approach is no longer advised, many patients arrived at their present high blood pressure treatment regimen by the stepwise approach and continue to take ineffective drugs along with the others.

When a patient comes to me asking for help in simplifying his blood pressure regimen, I will usually have the patient wean off the first antihypertension drug prescribed while monitoring blood pressure daily at home. At a follow-up visit, if the pressure has risen, the medicine is reinstated, and we repeat the process for the next drug. If blood pressure remains controlled without the drug, however, it is removed from the treatment permanently. Invariably, we find that the most recently added medications are doing the job, while the initially prescribed drugs are doing little. Often one or more medicines can be discontinued, allowing the patient to save money and clear some room in the medicine cabinet.

Management of hypertension can be quite complex, and you should not be too skeptical about how your treatment was determined. I only give these anecdotes as examples of inefficient prescribing, and offer ways to address the problem. In stepwise therapy, it is entirely appropriate to continue medicines that improve high blood pressure even if they do not bring it completely down to goal. This is usually the case for adding a second medicine, rather than making a substitution. Sometimes, a medicine doing little to lower blood pressure on its own will potentiate the effect of another. *Therefore, do not experiment with stopping blood pressure medicines or alter treatment in any way on your own—this could result in a rebound of dangerously high pressure! Make adjustments to therapy only with the guidance of your physician.*

What's This One Do Again?

It does pay to be attentive to the effectiveness of newly prescribed medicines. If you are given a new medication for the treatment of diabetes, you should see an improvement in blood sugar levels. A new cholesterol agent should lower your cholesterol. Did your anxiety resolve on the Lexapro? If there is no improvement, why should you continue buying and taking it? There have been some wonderful breakthroughs in the management of all these conditions, but medications do not work in every case, and many are quite expensive. If you do not see any benefit from a new treatment, ask your doctor if there is an appropriate substitution, rather than just adding on yet another costly agent.

There has been tremendous marketing to doctors and the public to treat Alzheimer disease patients with drugs that are of marginal benefit, but expensive nonetheless. Taking advantage of the desperate situation of these patients and their families is as ugly as the drug business gets. Anyone with a family member taking the drug Aricept (donepezil) should know that a study published in the *Lancet* in 2004 concluded that the drug does *not* improve behavioral or psychological symptoms. It does not affect progression of disability or delay admission to a nursing home. It does not prolong life or prevent adverse events. It has not been shown to help the psychological well-being of the caregiver, and it does not reduce overall treatment costs.[11] Patients treated in clinical trials initially do perform better on mental status exams and in activities of daily living. But after six months, their performance declines at the same rate as that of untreated patients. It is difficult to fault families (or physicians) for wanting to try some type of therapy targeted at helping their loved ones with Alzheimer's disease. But if minimal or no benefit is seen, the drug should be discontinued, and the $621 for three months' therapy saved.

Besides the drugs that don't work, get rid of the ones that can kill you. Some drugs used frequently in treating the agitation of Alzheimer's disease are associated with a higher risk of death! The FDA reported that, in *seventeen* randomized controlled trials, elderly dementia patients treated with the second-generation antipsychotics Abilify, Risperdal, Seroquel, and Zyprexa had a higher mortality rate than those receiving placebo.[12] Most of the deaths were due to strokes, blood clots, and infections such as pneumonia. This news is even more alarming when you consider that there is limited proof that these drugs help these patients. A recent systematic review found little evidence of clinical effectiveness for antipsychotic medications in dementia in general.[13] Now add the fact that the average retail price for ninety days' therapy with these drugs ranges from $483 for Seroquel to $1,365 for Abilify, and it really gets irritating. If you are not absolutely convinced of the essential benefit of one of these drugs for the treatment of agitated dementia, the drug should be stopped. You will save money and perhaps prevent unnecessary suffering and death.

One of the most heavily marketed and prescribed drugs for the treatment of asthma likewise has been shown to *increase* mortality from asthma. You read that right, salmeterol (one of the two drugs comprising the popular and expensive asthma treatment, Advair) was shown in a large study to increase the probability of asthma-related death in patients treated with this medication.[14] In this case, however, it is *not* that salmeterol is ineffective for treatment of symptoms associated with asthma; it is effective. It is just that there is a higher rate of death associated with its use. Since doctors in general are in the business of preserving life, I am not sure how any of us can justify initiating treatment of asthma with this drug. Short-acting bronchodilators and inhaled corticosteroids should be used first, and long-acting bronchodilators, like salmeterol, added only if absolutely needed. The FDA issued an Alert for Healthcare Professionals regarding Advair in July 2006, which states, "[I]n the treatment of asthma, Advair Diskus should only be used in patients who have not adequately responded to other asthma controller medications."[15]

Case Study
CSM 3: Eliminate Medicines That Have Never Worked

Henrietta is an eighty-four-year-old woman with Alzheimer's dementia. As her disease progressed, her daughter placed her in a board-and-care facility. The daughter remained attentive, visiting her mother daily and bringing her into the office for frequent assessments. With the confirmation of her illness,

Henrietta was given a trial of Aricept, but little benefit was seen. Consultation with the neurologist led to the addition of Namenda to the treatment regimen. After several months of the dual therapy, I met with Henrietta, her daughter, and her daily care provider to discuss her progress. The consensus was that no obvious benefit was seen with either of the drugs, and concern was expressed about the $1,159 price tag for three months' therapy. Her daughter told me that once her mother's financial resources were exhausted, transfer to a Medicaid nursing home would be the only option. We agreed to a trial discontinuation of both drugs. At follow-up, no drop in performance was reported and no change in mental status was noted. We agreed to keep Henrietta's treatment with medications as simple as possible, without further use of Aricept or Namenda. As of this writing, she continues to be well treated at the board-and-care home, without the burden of medications that never worked.

Yearly Savings: $4,636

CSM 4: Eliminate Medicines That Were Never Needed

So you're taking medicine to lower your blood pressure. Do you even have hypertension? "Sure, my pressure was 'a little high' just before they wheeled me in for a prostate biopsy, and I've been on medication ever since."

To be officially diagnosed with hypertension, a person must have two or more elevated blood pressure readings on two or more separate occasions. But before *I* get treated, I want far more readings than that, and not all of them in a scary doctor's office! The "white-coat syndrome" refers to artificially elevated blood pressure when taken by a health care professional (the white-coat) in a medical facility such as a hospital, office, or clinic. The spurious readings are probably due to a release of adrenaline in response to stress. A study using ambulatory blood pressure monitoring of patients under treatment at a university hospital hypertension clinic found that 25 percent of the patients did not even have hypertension! That's right—the original diagnosis was incorrect in one-fourth of the patients.[16]

The Cure for Which There Is No Disease

Too many new patients coming to me taking cholesterol drugs for primary prevention do not show appropriate criteria for such treatment in their records. Elevated total cholesterol as the sole rationale is inadequate. Some of these patients have pretreatment HDL ("good") cholesterol higher than their LDL ("bad") cholesterol, with total/HDL ratios putting them at less than half the standard risk for coronary heart disease. A sixty-eight-year-old woman taking Lipitor per her previous doctor's recommendation came to me for help. After trial discontinuation of the drug, we calculated her overall risk of cardiovascular disease for the next ten years at only 2 percent. That's a one in fifty chance that she would develop coronary heart disease by age seventy-eight! Then why the Lipitor?

Treatment of hypertension and high cholesterol is paramount in stroke and heart attack prevention, and it should be taken very seriously. But unjustified treatment for incorrect or unsubstantiated diagnoses does not help the cause, and it wastes health care dollars. I encourage patients to learn as much as possible about their conditions, both diagnosis and treatment, and get involved in their care. Challenge your doctor with questions and suggestions. Be sure you have adequate confirmation for every diagnosis and justification for treatment with medication. This may require multiple blood pressure readings measured at home or in the workplace, or serial cholesterol determinations including HDL and LDL together with an assessment of your overall cardiovascular disease risk status. You will get better care, and you may avoid a treatment for which there is no disease.

Case Study
CSM 4: Eliminate Medicines That Were Never Needed

Danielle is a fifty-year-old female teacher's aid who was called by her gynecologist's office staff with screening blood test results and told to begin taking Lipitor for high cholesterol. We reviewed the test results several months later. Her total and HDL cholesterol levels were 232 and 67, corresponding to a ratio of 3.5. LDL cholesterol was 146 and triglycerides were 93. The Coronary Heart Disease Risk chart on her lab reporting sheet indicated her risk to be at "half the standard risk." Going a step further, I plugged these numbers and other data (blood pressure, smoking status, and so on) into the risk calculator on the NCEP website (see chapter 4). Her ten-year risk for development of cardiovascular disease was calculated to be less than 1 percent. By questioning the therapy, Danielle found out that she was not at increased risk for coronary heart disease, that the recommendation for drug treatment was incorrect, and that she could eliminate a medicine that was never needed.

Yearly Savings: $1,192

Take It to the Bank

Find out the answers to these questions at your treatment review visit:

- What was the original indication for each medication? You absolutely must know why each drug was first prescribed. What was the diagnosis or problem, and how was it confirmed?
- Is each problem still active, and is ongoing therapy with drugs still warranted?
- Has each medication proven itself effective, and is each still effective at the present time?
- If there is any uncertainty about a medicine's effectiveness, is a trial discontinuation justified?
- For any medications that were started while you were in the hospital, what were the circumstances? Is continuing therapy still warranted?
- Are any medications feeding a habituation or simply taken to treat or prevent withdrawal symptoms?

You deserve answers to each of these questions, and your physician must be able to provide them. Your medical records should contain justification for treatment with all medications and documentation of the effectiveness of each. If your present doctor did not originally prescribe a medication, he must still be able to justify ongoing therapy. Perhaps medical records from a hospital or former doctor will elucidate. If not, challenge the therapy, and start eliminating those unnecessary expensive drugs.

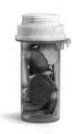

4

Think Outside the Prescription Drug Bottle

Cost-Saving Methods 5 through 7

AFTER ELIMINATING DRUGS YOU DON'T NEED, the best way to save money on prescription drugs is not to use them. I am not implying that you ignore your medical problems in order to save money on medications. (Although as we have seen, that tactic is used by many patients.) What I am saying is: whenever and as much as possible, use proven nonpharmacological methods to treat your medical problems instead of prescription drugs.

A Pill for Every Problem

Both doctors and patients have been sold on the notion that there is a pill for every problem. Do you have heartburn? Then take Prevacid. Do your joints ache? Get some Celebrex. Is work stressing you? Xanax will help. Can't sleep? Try Lunesta. Can't perform like you used to? Viagra! Depressed over how many drugs you take? Lexapro to the rescue!

Writing prescriptions is too easy for physicians. The act is symbolic of the end of the office visit. You know it is soon time to go when the doctor's pen is poised over a prescription pad. Physicians want patients to feel validated at their visits. This includes acknowledging problems and developing a treatment plan. But too often, the only plan is another trip to the pharmacy. Prescribing a drug has replaced comprehensive medical advice. A recent study reported that doctors only provide appropriate counseling to patients 18 percent of the time.[1]

Patients are equally to blame. They expect that taking a pill is all that is required to cure their ailments. When presented with a treatment program including lifestyle changes, the more encompassing recommendations are frequently left undone. Recommendations for modifications in diet and exercise are ignored, putting greater emphasis on drugs to achieve treatment goals. Physicians jump right to drug therapy, too, knowing there is little chance that patients will change old habits.

Please don't misunderstand me. I am not against prescription drugs. Medicines have done wonders to cure disease and improve health. Medications are indispensable tools. But drugs are not the only means of treatment, and for chronic problems, they are rarely the single best remedy. A return to the basic tenets of therapy is essential as drugs become increasingly expensive, to the point of being unaffordable to many.

CSM 5: Treat with Lifestyle Changes

Unless you have an exceptional doctor, having your medical problems addressed from a nonpharmacological perspective is going to take some added effort. You will need to push for more information and resources on treating effectively with a minimum of drugs. Similarly, the burden will fall squarely on you to comply with therapies requiring far more effort than simply swallowing a pill—therapies that could demand a complete restructuring of lifelong habits. A patient diagnosed with diabetes may be started on medication, but first he should be counseled on diet, exercise, health maintenance, and disease prevention. He should also be referred to a dietician or diabetes educator. The goal is to achieve and maintain control of the condition with as little medication as possible. Sadly, not only do few patients comply with the requisite lifestyle changes, but most never even bother to see the diabetes educator or learn the American Diabetes Association diet. They continue to eat and live as they always have, resigned to take several drugs for blood sugar control. Many will even submit to multiple daily insulin injections rather than lose a pound or walk an extra block.

Just Say No to Drugs

Want to save money on prescription drugs? Then learn how to manage your medical problems with less reliance on them. Instead of asking your doctor about a new medicine you see advertised on TV, you should be asking, "Isn't there a way to treat my problem without drugs?" Your condition may require medication at the outset, and your doctor will certainly inform you of this. But lifestyle changes are more likely to be prescribed if you ask about them. Compliance with therapy is then up to you.

Yes, Prevacid works wonders for treatment of heartburn caused by gastro-esophageal reflux disease (GERD) but so can reduction of caffeine, nicotine, and alcohol. GERD patients should avoid overeating, should not eat within two hours of bedtime, and should lose weight if necessary. The health benefits of these measures will be far greater than any realized by just taking a pill. Such lifestyle changes might add years to your life. But even if the only lifestyle change is raising the head of your bed by six inches, it could save you $2,228 per year*–well worth the effort.

No one can argue that anti-inflammatory medications including the newer Cox II inhibitors (e.g., Celebrex) have not been of great benefit to sufferers of arthritis and other musculoskeletal ailments. But with the recent withdrawal of Vioxx from the market and scares surrounding related drugs, many patients began looking for alternative treatments. It has been amazing how many who once relied on these drugs are now managing quite well with exercise, yoga, or physical therapy. It is embarrassing how few were previously offered any treatment modality other than prescription drugs.

* Average retail cost of one year's therapy with daily Prevacid.

"Great, Doc, but I have high blood pressure. Drugs are the only way for me."

Wrong! According to the National Institutes of Health, "Adoption of healthy lifestyles . . . is an indispensable part of the management of those with hypertension."[2] Weight reduction in overweight and obese individuals significantly lowers blood pressure. The Trials of Hypertension, Phase II study showed a five- to twenty-point drop in systolic blood pressure with each twenty-two pounds of weight loss. Overweight individuals may be only twenty pounds away from a twenty-point reduction in blood pressure, without prescription drugs. Adoption of the DASH eating plan* lowers systolic blood pressure by eight to fourteen points. Include a low-salt diet, and the effect is similar to single-drug therapy. Regular aerobic physical activity such as brisk walking thirty minutes per day, and moderation of alcohol consumption to less than two beverages per day, reduces systolic blood pressure by an additional six to thirteen points, all without popping a single pill![3]

High cholesterol should also first be treated with diet. A strict low-fat diet was shown in a clinical study to lower triglycerides, and both total and LDL cholesterol, as much as "statin" drugs (such as Crestor, Lescol, Lipitor, Pravachol, Zocor, and the like).[4] The same study found that *over half* of the doctors of the patients enrolled had not prescribed dietary therapy before initiating drugs! With today's stricter guidelines for optimal cholesterol levels, especially for those with diabetes or known

---

* The DASH eating plan is rich in fruits, vegetables, and low-fat dairy products, with a reduced content of saturated and total fat.

vascular disease, diet may not be enough. But it stands to reason that the better the diet, the less medication will be needed to reach treatment goals, and the less money will be spent on prescription drugs.

Case Study
CSM 5: Treat with Lifestyle Changes

Ernesto is a forty-nine-year-old dentist who developed diabetes in 1999. Fasting blood sugar was elevated at 190 (normal: 70–110), and glycohemoglobin (an index of average blood sugar over a three-month period) was also high at 8.5 (normal: 4.5–5.7). He weighed 242 pounds and did not adhere to any particular diet or exercise program.

Ernesto's treatment of diabetes began with a consultation with a registered dietician for counseling on diet and weight reduction. Within the first ten pounds of weight loss, Ernesto's blood sugar measurements improved. By three months, he had achieved our treatment goal of glycohemoglobin below 7 percent. Over the next six years, his weight was maintained at between 215 and 225 pounds, and his blood sugar remained strictly controlled without medication. As of this writing, his diabetes is not even detectable by fasting blood sugar or glycohemoglobin.

Pharmacy Cost (for six years of optimal diabetes management)**: $0.00**

CSM 6: Use Nondrug Treatments

Say you've done all you can to adopt healthy changes in lifestyle, but your medical problems are still not under control. Next stop, the prescription drug counter, right? Not necessarily. I shouldn't have to tell you that there are a multitude of therapies out there besides prescription drugs. Some are well within the mainstream of Western medicine, such as physical therapy, physical rehabilitation, psychotherapy, surgery, and chronic pain management. Most doctors commonly refer patients for these services. Other treatment modalities are a little more on the fringe of Western medicine, such as hypnosis, yoga, and acupuncture. Fewer doctors refer patients for these services. Many approaches to healing fall into the category of "alternative medicine," meaning outside the realm of traditional Western medicine.

There may be any number of reasons that you might prefer a nondrug approach to the treatment of your medical problems. But first let me say that these therapies may not necessarily be cheaper than prescription drugs. Some may be quite expensive and may not be covered by your health insurance plan. A lot more than cost should weigh into how best to manage your care, but the objective here is to make your treatment affordable.

Get *Proven* Relief

If you are looking for advice on medical therapies outside of traditional Western medicine, this isn't your book. Don't get me wrong; I'm for anything that works. But you have to prove to me that it works, safely, consistently, and for most people under similar circumstances. Any proposed therapy should have clinical studies to back it, confirmed with modern statistical analysis. Otherwise, it is not worth your time and money. (This includes prescription drugs.) A news story won't cut it, nor will a book, website, or newspaper advice column, even if written by an MD. There are charlatans in every profession, and medicine is no exception. Everything from ancient Andean remedies to miracle cure-alls is marketed to a hopeful and gullible public. The limitations and high costs of Western medicine fuel faith in these dubious restoratives. Some of these cures may have merit, but most have not been subject to the testing standards of modern medicine. When patients ask me about an unorthodox therapy, if I don't know of any clinical studies to support it, I cannot condone it. The treatment could be helpful, or it could do nothing. It may even be harmful, so experimenting with a treatment based on marketing claims or testimonials is not prudent.

The placebo-controlled, randomized, double-blind, peer-reviewed clinical trial with statistical analysis has become the standard means of justifying a therapy in Western medicine. *Placebo-controlled* means that the treatment group is measured against similar patients who do not receive the treatment. In a clinical trial of a new drug, for example, the effect of the drug in a treatment group is compared to a like group receiving an unmedicated preparation (the placebo). You can't say a treatment is effective if you don't compare it to what happens without the treatment. *Randomized* means that patients are divided into the treatment and placebo groups by chance, or at random. This guards against a potential bias in dividing up the treatment groups. *Double blind* means that neither the researchers nor the patients know who is receiving the treatment and who is getting the placebo until the trial is completed. This also serves to filter out bias in assessing the benefits and side effects of the treatment, by doctors or patients. The results of the study must then undergo analysis to make sure they reach statistical significance. This determines the probability that the findings are accurate. The greater the number of patients enrolled in the study, the more likely the results are valid. You should always be skeptical of treatment results reported on small numbers of patients. This is especially true of personal testimonials. A single person claiming to be cured or helped by any type of treatment (even your favorite aunt) is not adequate proof that the therapy is likely to be effective for most other people. *Peer reviewed* means that the results are examined by other, uninvolved researchers with an objective eye. Finally, a trustworthy study should not be funded by commercial interests, and the authors should not have financial ties to the company that makes the drug being tested.[5] This type of study is the gold standard of medical research. If a treatment is shown to be effective under these conditions, it is likely to be beneficial for you.

Valuable information is also obtained from observational studies. These studies collect information about large numbers of people observed over a long period of time. Statistics are used to correlate all manner of data with all manner of outcomes. The observation that women who take estrogen after menopause have a higher incidence of stroke, but a lower incidence of hip fractures than untreated women, is one example.[6]

So why don't all types of treatments, from ancient potions to Eastern remedies to new alternative therapies, undergo this type of scrutiny? It might be very interesting, revealing some marvelous cures and debunking frivolous remedies. Why doesn't somebody just go ahead and perform some clinical trials on this stuff? You might want to ask the people doing the studies. Commercial interests sponsor much of the medical research these days. There's no money in testing treatments you cannot patent and sell, and the drug manufacturers don't see any reason to give these treatments any additional competition-producing credibility. Likewise, marketers of newfangled snake oil elixirs have little to gain by honestly testing their products. Why would they want to risk showing that a cleverly marketed and profitable product is in fact no better than a placebo? So whom can we trust?

I still believe that the practice of medicine is an art, but it has a basis in science. In that tradition, any proposed therapy must be validated by legitimate clinical trials as described above. Where that is not possible, the available data should be extrapolated to make reasonable treatment recommendations. That is not to say that Western medicine has never erred using this approach. The blanket recommendation for hormone replacement therapy (HRT) for most postmenopausal women endorsed by the medical profession in the last two decades remains an embarrassment.* But Western medicine is usually

---

* HRT was shown to increase breast cancer, heart attack, stroke, and blood clots by the Women's Health Initiative.[7]

honest in its successes and failures, and I only want to steer you toward treatments that are very likely to be successful.

Prescription Alternatives

Clearly, volumes could be written on all of the nonpharmacological therapies available. My intention here is to give you but a few examples of evidence-based nondrug treatments that are direct alternatives to popular expensive prescription drugs. The idea is to encourage you to remind your doctor that for many conditions, prescription drugs are not the only valid alternative. Once you get the idea, you can research and discuss alternative treatments for your medical problems with your doctor.

Epley Procedure for Vertigo

Benign Positional Vertigo (BPV) is a common disorder characterized by recurrent dizziness brought on by movement. It is caused by the formation of crystals in the inner ear. Phenergan, Bonine, and Ativan are some drugs used to treat BPV. All of them are sedating; none are cures. They primarily mask symptoms while the patient waits for the condition to improve. But there is a cure for BPV that is not a drug. A series of therapeutic maneuvers called the Epley procedure was developed, which can displace the offending crystals. German researchers published a study wherein patients used video instruction of the Epley procedure to treat BPV at home. After one week, vertigo was abolished in 95 percent of the patients. No medications were required.[8]

Yoga for Low-Back Pain

The effectiveness of yoga for treatment of patients with chronic low-back pain was proven in a clinical trial published in the *Annals of Internal Medicine*.[9] Patients with up to fifteen months of back pain were randomized to receive either three months of weekly yoga classes, three months of exercise classes, or self-care books. At three months, the yoga group had significantly less disability than the other groups. At six months, not only did the benefits continue, but the yoga participants also reported *significantly less medication use* for back pain than did patients in the other groups.

Cognitive-Behavioral Therapy for Anxiety

Several randomized clinical trials have shown that cognitive-behavioral therapy (a type of psychological counseling) is as effective as tranquillizers or antidepressants for treatment of anxiety disorders. The benefit lasts or even increases following completion of the therapy, with no ongoing costs and no medication side effects.[10]

Case Study
CSM 6: Use Nondrug Treatments

Inez is a fifty-one-year-old female martial arts teacher with migraine headaches. With menopause, her headaches became more frequent and difficult to manage. They began to occur daily for periods of time, starting behind the right eye, spreading into the sinuses, then into the neck and right shoulder. The migraine drug Imitrex was effective, but headaches often returned after six to eight hours. Consultation with a neurologist led to the addition of Topamax. The frequency of her headaches lessened, but the two migraine drugs were running over $400 per month.

Inez began a program of physical therapy for neck and shoulder spasms and learned stress-reduction techniques. After five weeks of therapy, she reported eighteen consecutive headache-free days (the most in over a year), and she was able to stop the Topamax. She switched to a home exercise program and had only one severe headache over the next three months. At six months she reported fewer, shorter, and less-severe headaches, managed with one or two Imitrex tablets per month.

Yearly Savings: $4,585

CSM 7: Prevent Disease Naturally

It is hard to deny that we are wasting lots of money on ineffective pills and elixirs for prevention of all manner of ills. We seem to prefer spending money trying to find medications to counter the effects of our bad habits, rather than changing the habits.

—Douglas Kamerow, US editor, *British Medical Journal*

I hope we can all agree that the best way to manage disease is to avoid getting sick in the first place. Disease prevention should be a top priority. Table 4-1 lists some major preventable health problems in the United States today. Fortunately, there are modifiable risk factors for each—things that can be identified and changed to prevent us from getting sick. Modifiable (and nonmodifiable) risk factors for these conditions are listed in tables 4-2 through 4-5.

Although these are a diverse group of diseases, a quick perusal of the modifiable risk factors identifies the same culprits over and over: cigarette smoking, sedentary lifestyle, high fat diet, and obesity. What a sorry list! Who wants to work on *those* issues to stay healthy? If only there was a pill we could take to prevent disease instead. But wait! High cholesterol is listed, and there's a pill for that. Forget all that other stuff; pass the Lipitor!

TABLE 4-1: Some Important Preventable Diseases

Heart attack, stroke, cancer, diabetes, hip fracture

TABLE 4-2: Risk Factors for Stroke and Heart Attack

Modifiable

Cigarette smoking, sedentary lifestyle (poor physical fitness), high blood pressure, high-fat "Western" diet, diabetes, high total or LDL cholesterol/ low HDL cholesterol/high triglycerides

Nonmodifiable

Family history, age (male over 45, female over 55)

TABLE 4-3: Risk Factors for Hip Fracture[11]

Modifiable

Low bone mineral density (osteoporosis), frailty/weakness/inactivity, medication side effects, visual impairment, cigarette smoking, alcoholism, propensity to falls, weight under 125 pounds

Nonmodifiable

Age over 80 (two thirds of hip-fracture victims), history of fracture after age 40, parental fracture after age 50, caucasian, female sex, dementia

TABLE 4-4: Risk Factors for Diabetes
Modifiable
Obesity, sedentary lifestyle
Nonmodifiable
Family history, age

TABLE 4-5: Risk Factors for Cancer
Modifiable
Sedentary lifestyle, cigarette smoking, high-fat "Western" diet, obesity
Nonmodifiable
Family history, age

A Pound of Prevention for an Ounce of Cure?

Should we spend money on drugs to reduce the chance that we might get a disease? This is an important question when it comes to affordability of prescription treatment. The top-selling drug in 2005, with over sixty-three million prescriptions written, was given primarily to *prevent* disease. That's right: the cholesterol-lowering drug Lipitor grossed more in sales than any other medicine, $11.36 billion.[12] The majority of those prescriptions were not to treat illness, but rather to reduce the chance of cardiovascular disease in people who had never had a stroke or heart attack. Let's clarify something here: The ultimate goal of taking Lipitor is *not* to lower your cholesterol level. You are prescribed Lipitor to reduce the chance that you will have a heart attack or stroke. Crestor, gemfibrozil, Lescol, lovastatin, Pravachol, Tricor, Vytorin, Zetia, and Zocor are other cholesterol treatments used primarily for prevention. That amounts to a huge sum of health care spending, money coming out of your pocket. Is it worth it? Well, it depends on the following factors:

1. The seriousness of the disease
2. *Your* likelihood of getting the disease
3. The effectiveness of medication in preventing the disease
4. What *else* you can do to lower the risk
5. If you can afford the medication

Number 1, *seriousness*, is obvious when it comes to any of the conditions in table 4-1; they are all serious. Number 2, *likelihood*, will vary depending on your age, gender, race, habits, diet, and other risk factors for the disease. Numbers 3, 4, and 5 combined constitute the value of the treatment. Is the expense of the medication worth its potential benefit compared to other ways of reducing disease risk? That will depend on your means, your motivation to adopt other preventive methods, and your tolerance for risk. It is not a one-size-fits-all proposition as the current, drug-driven medical culture dictates. Let's look at these factors in regard to cardiovascular disease.

Heart Disease: What Are the Chances?

Thanks to the Framingham Heart Study, your risk of developing coronary heart disease (CHD) can be simply and accurately predicted.[13] The Framingham assessment weighs not just cholesterol but also multiple risk factors to predict the chances of developing CHD. Your doctor should be able to calculate your risk for you. If not, you can easily do it yourself using the "risk assessment tool" on the National Cholesterol

Education Program (NCEP) website.* Just plug in the seven data points including age, sex, total and HDL cholesterol, blood pressure, and smoking history. Then click the "Calculate ten-year risk" button. If your risk for CHD for the next ten years is greater than 10 to 20 percent, you should seriously consider the value of preventive therapy with cholesterol drugs. Drug treatment for those with risk below 10 percent is usually not needed. Nevertheless, it is troubling how many people with a ten-year risk assessment of only a few percentage points or less are currently paying for cholesterol drugs at the recommendation of their doctors.

Cholesterol Drugs: How Much Protection?

How effective are cholesterol drugs in preventing cardiovascular disease, anyway? Studies consistently report a 30 to 40 percent relative risk reduction in heart disease in healthy patients taking these drugs.[14] This sounds impressive, but the concept of *relative risk* can be misleading. The relative risk relates to the difference between test groups. But how much would treatment lower *your* risk under similar circumstances? It wouldn't be 40 percent. The reduction in new disease in relation to the total number of people treated is the "absolute risk reduction," a more practical measure of the effectiveness of a treatment. For example, a landmark study supporting preventive treatment showed that the absolute risk reduction of taking lovastatin for 5.2 years was only 2 percent.[15] In other words, one hundred people (under similar circumstances)

* Go to http://hin.nhlbi.nih.gov/atpiii/calculator.asp?usertype=prof, or type "NCEP CVD risk" into any search engine.

would have to take lovastatin for five years to prevent two serious heart events. The cost per person of that preventive treatment is about $8,320* for drugs alone. The brand name Zocor would cost $10,644. If your doctor said to you, "You're in good health, but your cholesterol is high; do you want to spend $8,000 to $10,000 on medicine over the next five years to reduce your chance of a first heart attack by 2 percent?" would you do it? Why isn't the decision to use this therapy presented in this way?

A study published in *The Lancet* in 2002 was even more sobering. For high-risk patients from age seventy to eighty-two *who did not already have vascular disease*, taking Pravachol (pravastatin) did not reduce the risk of heart disease or stroke at all![16] The Cardiovascular Health Study, published in the *Journal of the American Geriatric Society* two years later, showed that, for people over 65, total and LDL cholesterol levels aren't even related to heart attack rates or overall mortality.[17] Those findings sure make it hard to justify primary preventive treatment in that age group, or even to justify screening the elderly for high cholesterol levels at all.

Protect Your Heart Naturally

How does lowering high cholesterol with drugs measure up with modifying other risk factors? Let's look at physical fitness. In a study of twenty-five thousand male executives who were followed for ten years, there were three times as many deaths due to strokes, heart attack, and blood clots in the men in the worst physical shape than there were in men

---

* The average retail price at 40 mg daily for 5.2 years.

with high cholesterol.[18] Those men who improved their fitness cut their risk of cardiovascular death by 50 percent! The Framingham Heart Study also showed that physical activity directly correlates with survival. The most-active third of the five thousand men and women studied had a 40 percent lower death rate than did the least-active third.[19] So being in poor physical shape is more dangerous than high cholesterol, and improving conditioning reduces mortality more than cholesterol drugs do.

Smoking is responsible for as much as 30 percent of all deaths from coronary heart disease.[20] It would seem that smoking cessation is a far more effective way to stay healthy than taking a medication to lower cholesterol. It is ironic how many people take cholesterol drugs while continuing to smoke cigarettes. Not only will quitting smoking prevent heart attacks and stroke better than an expensive cholesterol drug would, it will also avert emphysema, chronic bronchitis, and cancers of the lung, mouth, esophagus, bladder, and larynx. *And* the savings on cigarettes, insurance rates, and prescriptions amount to thousands of dollars per year.

Can diet prevent deaths due to coronary heart disease? A landmark study published in the *British Medical Journal* in 2005 showed that elderly Europeans eating a modified Mediterranean diet reduced their rate of death due to *all* causes by up to 12 percent.[21] Several other studies have also shown a correlation between this diet and increased survival.[22] The Mediterranean diet is high in vegetables, fruits, grains, fish, and unsaturated fats (particularly olive oil). It is low in meat, dairy products, and saturated fats and includes a moderate intake of alcohol, mostly in the form of wine. Sounds like a much more palatable way to improve survival than taking a cholesterol pill!

The reduction in *first* heart attacks by cholesterol drugs is actually quite modest compared to lifestyle changes. A worldwide study published in the journal *Lancet* found that a combination of healthful diet, regular exercise, and smoking cessation reduced the risk of a first heart attack by a staggering 81 percent![23] Furthermore, taking a cholesterol pill does nothing to lower weight, increase fitness, improve vitality, or walk the dog like exercise can. So if you can't afford a drug-based prevention program, you might want to go with lifestyle changes, including exercise. (I'm pretty sure I know which one your dog wants you to choose!)

Let me emphasize that I am talking about *primary prevention*: stopping the development of disease in otherwise healthy people. The case for treatment of high cholesterol in persons who already have cardiovascular disease (secondary prevention), or who are at highest risk, is much more compelling (unless you're over eighty—in that group, statins have not been shown to prolong life, even when given immediately following a new heart attack[24]).

Those patients whose doctors follow NCEP guidelines in treating to bring LDL cholesterol to very low levels (below 70 mg/dl) for secondary prevention should know that a recent review of all available data (including the studies used by the NCEP) did not find solid evidence to support the necessity of achieving these low levels. Greater decreases in LDL cholesterol were not associated with fewer recurrent heart attacks than smaller reductions.[25] But such treatment is riskier and usually more expensive.

Cholesterol in Perspective

In view of the high cost of statins, it is time that the true value of these drugs in the primary prevention of CHD be presented frankly to the consumer. If your doctor only says, "Your cholesterol is high; start taking Lipitor," you have not been well served. The cost of this therapy does not permit a blanket recommendation for all patients on the basis of cholesterol level alone. The ability of cholesterol drugs to prevent disease should be presented honestly and applied to the individual, in consideration of his or her risk. Factors including blood pressure, diabetes, smoking, diet, exercise, family history, weight, belief in drug-based prevention, and *means* should be reviewed. Then let the patient decide just how much insurance against disease he or she wants to buy. There may also be an unrealistic expectation of what these drugs can do—not in lowering cholesterol levels, which is usually impressive, but in *preventing disease*. You have a right to know just how effective a preventive drug treatment is likely to be and how much it costs. Then *you* decide if you want to buy it.

There is also another drug that lowers the probability of cardiovascular disease for patients at high risk. It is much more cost effective than any cholesterol pill. Results of clinical trials show up to a 34 percent reduction in heart attack in men and a 25 percent reduction in stroke in women taking this miracle drug just once a day.[26] And it's dirt cheap; a year of treatment costs less than ten bucks! The drug? Aspirin. Unfortunately, aspirin also increases the risk of bleeding, primarily from the stomach and intestinal tract, and also the risk of bleeding strokes. Still, the risk-to-benefit ratio is favorable for those at highest risk of CHD. So for primary prevention of heart attack and stroke in high-risk individuals over age fifty, aspirin may be an inexpensive option.

Due in large part to our friends in the pharmaceutical industry, cholesterol control has become the main focus of preventive health care in the United States. But what about more important prevention measures? Instead of asking, "What's your cholesterol?" it would make more sense to ask, "How many miles do you walk per week?" or "How much have you cut animal products out of your diet?" or, better yet, "Have you quit smoking yet?" The answers to these questions will give you a better indication of the person's overall risk of health problems than his or her cholesterol level will.

Preoccupation with cholesterol has distracted both doctor and patient from a more comprehensive discussion of preventive health care. If your doctor determines that you may be headed for serious health problems, *all* of the modifiable risk factors should be discussed. Identify where changes in diet, exercise, weight, and lifestyle can be made, and start preventing disease naturally!

Case Study
CSM 7: **Prevent Disease Naturally**

Kent is a sixty-two-year-old retired computer programmer taking Crestor for high cholesterol, prescribed by a prior physician. He had never had heart disease, his average systolic blood pressure was 124 without medication, and he had never smoked. At the time of our first consultation, he was not exercising regularly nor observing any particular diet. Records showed a total cholesterol of 242 before treatment with Crestor and 204 after. He seemed pleased with these results—a 38-point drop in total cholesterol. The only problem was the $354 cost for three months of medication.

To help Kent understand the risk reduction of his treatment, I plugged his cholesterol values and other pertinent data into the risk calculation program on the NCEP website.* According to the risk calculator, before treatment with Crestor, his risk of developing heart disease over the next ten years was 12 percent. Entering the posttreatment values, his risk was 10 percent.

Although Kent's total cholesterol improved nicely with the Crestor, he was not impressed with the 2 percent reduction in his ten-year risk assessment, especially considering the cost of the medication. We discussed other methods of cardiovascular risk reduction and lowering cholesterol. He decided to stop taking Crestor, reduce intake of animal fats, and begin an exercise program. Within three months, Kent's total and HDL cholesterol levels were 202 and 51. This corresponded to a new ten-year risk assessment of 9 percent, slightly better than that obtained with Crestor alone.

Yearly Savings: $1,416

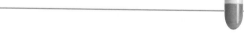

* http://hin.nhlbi.nih.gov/atpiii/calculator.asp?usertype=prof

Hip Fractures: What Are the Chances?

Expensive medicines are also widely prescribed to prevent hip fractures due to osteoporosis. Fosamax was already in the top thirty most-prescribed drugs in 2004, with over twenty million prescriptions written. Actonel, Boniva, Evista, and Miacalcin are not far behind. A year of preventive therapy with any of these drugs is about $1,200. Is it worth it? Again, it depends upon your risk, the potential of the drug, and what else you can do to prevent fractures.

Bone mineral density (BMD) is but one factor in determining fracture risk. Nonetheless, measuring BMD by DEXA and other scans to calculate a T-score is now the primary means of assessing fracture risk in the United States. Recommendation for drug therapy often follows, sometimes on the test-results reporting sheet itself. However, the decision to take an osteoporosis drug should not be based on T-score alone. This results in prescribing to a great many women at low risk. Treatment should be individualized to overall risk: the number and severity of *all* risk factors.

Internet-savvy readers can access an excellent website that allows you to calculate your risk of hip fracture over the next ten years.* It is a risk-assessment tool developed by the World Health Organization called FRAX that integrates multiple clinical risk factors for fracture. From the home page, click on your ethnic background under the "calculation tool" heading, and then enter the twelve data points including femoral neck or total hip BMD. Using patient models from worldwide

* Go to www.shef.ac.uk/FRAX/index.htm, or type "WHO FRAX" into any search engine.

studies, your ten-year probability for hip fracture will be determined. Recommendations for treatment are not given, since, according to the website, "treatment will depend upon the costs of intervention, [and] the wealth of the individual. . . ."[27]

Osteoporosis Drugs: How Much Protection?

Unless you have already had a fracture due to osteoporosis, drugs are not very effective in preventing hip fractures. The Fracture Intervention Trial showed no significant reduction in hip fractures after four years of Fosamax for women without prior vertebral (backbone) fractures.* Another four-year study of over 4,200 women with low BMD treated with Fosamax showed a reduction in hip fractures from 1.1 percent to 0.9 percent.[28] That equates to two fewer hip fractures per one thousand women treated for four years. The cost of four years of therapy with Fosamax for one thousand women amounts to $4.9 million for drugs alone. That's $4.9 million spent, 2 fractures prevented. Not too impressive. In the largest Actonel study, osteoporotic women who did not have preexisting vertebral fractures saw no reduction in hip fractures after three years.[29] A three-year study on the newest osteoporosis drug, Boniva, showed the incidence of nonvertebral fractures, including hip fractures, was *higher* with Boniva than in the placebo group![30]

Evista (raloxifene) belongs to a different class of drugs to treat osteoporosis, but it has not been shown to prevent hip fractures (although it does increase the risk of fatal blood

---

* According to the Fosamax prescribing information in the package insert.

clots). Likewise, Miacalcin (calcitonin) has not been associated with significant reductions in fractures other than vertebral ones. Of course there's nothing wrong with reducing vertebral fractures, but hip fractures account for most of the costs, infirmity, and deaths attributed to osteoporosis. It's not fair to scare otherwise healthy women with statistics about the devastation of hip fractures in order to promote drugs that primarily reduce the risk of vertebral fractures.

Save Your Bones Naturally

What else is there, then? Well, remember that low bone-mineral density (BMD) is only one of the modifiable risk factors for hip fractures. Inactivity is another. Several large studies show a 33 to 55 percent reduction in hip fractures in the most active women.[31] So if your goal is to reduce the risk of hip fractures, a few hours of exercise each week, even walking, will do it better than expensive drugs. You also get all the other added benefits of exercise, and the cost at the drugstore is zero.

Taking calcium and vitamin D has been shown to reduce fracture rates, including hip fractures, in some studies by 22 to 33 percent, without side effects.[32] (Fosamax and Actonel can't claim that!) A three-month supply of combination calcium and vitamin D in therapeutic doses costs as little as $6.49. Although limited to only one study, inexpensive supplements of folic acid and mecobalamin (the bioactive form of vitamin B12) reduced the risk of osteoporotic hip fractures in stroke victims by 22 percent.[33] There is now evidence that a diet higher in vegetable than animal protein also reduces the risk of osteoporotic fractures.[34]

Several studies show a significant reduction in hip fractures in nursing home residents who wear hip protectors.[35] A study from Sweden demonstrated a reduction in fractures in nursing home patients undergoing risk assessment and intervention to prevent falls.[36] Makes more sense than giving them all another pill, doesn't it?

Summary

If sufficient resources are available to offer all patients every proven preventive health measure, fine. Let's send everybody to the health club and the dietician, and feed them Lipitor and Fosamax too. But, as the National Osteoporosis Foundation states on its website, "Some effective therapeutic options that would be prohibitively expensive on a population basis might remain a valid choice in individual cases."[37] I take this to mean that not everybody is going to be able to afford preventive drugs. For those with limited means who must foot the bill for their prescription drugs, some hard choices have to be made. I assume that if you are reading this book, you or someone close to you is strapped by prescription drug costs. It is for these folks that I recommend using medications first for treatment of actual medical conditions. Treat the diseases you have now. Next, use proven nondrug means to stay healthy and to prevent serious diseases you don't have. Only then should you consider the value of buying prescription drugs for further disease prevention. This will depend on your means and how much risk you are willing to accept. The following chapters and cost-saving methods will outline ways that may enable you to obtain even preventive treatments with prescription drugs if you decide you want to take them.

Take It to the Bank

- Always ask your doctor how you can treat your medical problems without prescription drugs. What changes in diet, activity level, tobacco use, alcohol consumption, or other lifestyle choices can be made?
- Inquire about nondrug treatments including physical therapy and rehabilitation, psychotherapy and counseling, surgical procedures, chronic pain management, acupuncture, yoga, and so on that have been proven effective by standard research methods.
- For disease prevention, use exercise, smoking cessation, improved diet, and blood pressure and diabetes control first. Consider adding drug therapy for prevention of disease only after obtaining all of the following:

    1. An accurate assessment of your risk of getting the disease
    2. Honest disclosure of the risk-reduction benefit of the drug
    3. Knowledge of the cost of the drug

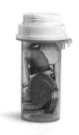

5

Steer Clear
of Overpriced
Redundant Drugs

Cost-Saving Methods
8 through 12

THE NEXT FIVE COST-SAVING METHODS (CSMs) allow you to
avoid or replace unnecessarily expensive treatments. That
might sound presumptuous—how could you possibly second-
guess the physician by declining a new prescription or suggesting substitutions for some on your present list? Isn't each drug
your doctor prescribes carefully selected for your particular
needs? Well, if you can't afford it, the answer is, "Obviously
not!" Remember, we physicians are out of touch with drug

costs, and it has fallen upon you, the consumers of health care, to challenge the status quo.

Before you can determine if a treatment is unnecessarily expensive, you must understand the distinction between "breakthrough" medicines and overpriced redundant drugs (ORDs). A breakthrough drug is an innovation in treatment. It is the first medication to effectively treat an illness or medical condition, or the first that provides a substantial improvement over existing therapies. A redundant drug just adds another choice to the pharmacist's shelf without any particular advantage, but often with a higher cost. You might think that all of the marvelous biomedical technology and research of today is yielding a steady stream of continuously superior drugs. Pharmaceutical advertising would certainly encourage you to think so. Even I marvel at the claims made in those ads. Each newly introduced product seems ever-improved over previous offerings, paving the way to better health and survival. Doctors must believe this too. Why else would we continually prescribe the latest—and costliest—drugs? Surely these new drugs represent therapeutic breakthroughs well worth their high prices.

Sorry to dispel the myth of modern drug therapy, but this just isn't true. Most of the new medicines patented every year are overpriced redundant drugs. They are new versions of old treatments. Many are not even as good as the drugs they are marketed to replace but are sold at many times the price. ORDs are the poorest values in drug therapy, but they account for over 40 percent of prescriptions.

Better Than Nothing?

In order to gain FDA approval, drug manufacturers only need to show that their product is superior to a placebo—that is, that it is better than no treatment at all. A new drug does not need to be tested against or shown to be superior to established medicines in use for the same treatment. But once it is approved, a marketing blitz for the product can drive popularity and sales. Billions of dollars are spent each year marketing redundant drugs to physicians and consumers, with insinuations that have little scientific basis. Doctors and patients have responded, helping establish record profits for an industry with a low rate of innovation.

In 2003, a group from the University of British Columbia determined that redundant drugs accounted for 44 percent of all prescriptions and 63 percent of total drug expenditures.[1] And that's in *Canada*, where there is better control of drug spending than in the United States! That's a large chunk of the prescription dollar for treatments that offer nothing extra besides aggressive marketing and a hefty price.

Too Many Reruns

So just how many new drugs represent legitimate breakthroughs, anyway? Fifty percent? Seventy-five percent? In her book, *The Truth about the Drug Companies*, former editor in chief of the *New England Journal of Medicine* Marcia Angell calculated that from 1998 to 2002, only 14 percent of drugs approved by the FDA showed significant improvement over existing medicines.[2] The Canadian Patented Prices Review

Board also appraised the therapeutic novelty of drugs intro-duced in Canada between 1990 and 2003. Most of these are the same drugs we have here, the ones many US citizens are buying cheaper from Canadian pharmacies. The board found that of 1,147 newly patented drugs, *less than 6 percent* provided a substantial improvement over less expensive existing medi-cines.[3] I cannot resist restating the obvious here: more than 94 percent of new drugs were found to be expensive remakes of treatments already in use. Thus the premise for the next few cost-saving methods: to keep prescription costs down, avoid or replace these costly, redundant products.

A simple way to avoid new treatment with an ORD is to steer clear of newer patented drugs. These are the ones adver-tised in the media and sent as samples to doctors' offices. The knowledge that about nine of ten new drugs are ORDs should be enough to convince you to *never* "ask your doctor" about any brand-name product you see advertised on TV (cost-saving method 8). You should also be wary of any new treatment started with samples provided to your doctor by the drug companies (cost-saving method 9). If you are already taking overpriced redundant drugs, cost-saving methods 10, 11, and 12 explain how to get affordable substitutions. These are also identified in the Expensive-Drug Survival Index.

There often isn't an equivalent alternative to a new break-through drug. Enbrel, for rheumatoid arthritis, is an example. You can either afford to buy it or not. But such drugs represent just a fraction of expensive, new products, and it's likely that other cost-saving methods will enable the therapy.

The good news is that by probability alone, it is very likely that an expensive drug you are taking is not a unique therapy, but is an ORD. There are probably multiple well-established medications available that serve the same purpose. Many of these may work as well or better for a much lower price. Many insurance prescription plans and pharmacy benefit managers (such as Caremark, Express Scripts, and Medco) are sending information and requests to doctors and patients outlining medication substitutions at a much lower cost. Recently, a patient showed me how changing her calcium channel blocker from Norvasc to generic felodipine, and her PPI from Protonix to omeprazole, would save her $369 per year through her prescription drug plan. I was happy to prescribe the cheaper medicines—which proved just as effective—at a nice savings to her. Read on to learn how you can avoid new prescriptions of overpriced redundant drugs, and how to suggest cheaper substitutions to your doctor for these unnecessarily expensive treatments.

CSM 8: Don't "Ask Your Doctor" (for Advertised Drugs)

If you want to save money on prescription drugs, one of the worst things you can do is to "ask your doctor" about medications you see advertised in the media. Those TV spots for prescription drugs are not public service announcements; they are advertisements like any others. In 1999 your representatives in the US Congress finalized legislation giving drug companies approval to advertise prescription drugs on television and in other media.[4] It is not an experiment by the pharmaceutical industry to see if such marketing might increase sales. It works. A report by the Kaiser Family Foundation states that heavily advertised direct-to-consumer (DTC) drugs are among the highest-grossing prescription drugs.[5] Is it any wonder that so many pharmaceutical advertisements are appearing on our televisions these days? Every other commercial seems to be promoting some new drug. Don't expect the trend to fade soon. The strategy has paid off so well that the drug companies have increased spending on DTC advertising to more than $4 billion per year.[6]

Is Spending a Fortune on Drugs Right for You?

By asking a doctor for a specific drug, you are more likely to receive it. If that doesn't sound intuitive enough for you, it was actually proven and reported in the *Journal of the American Medical Association* (*JAMA*) in April of 2005.[7] If a company can convince you to ask for their drug by name, the chance of a sale skyrockets by more than tenfold! The same study also showed that patients requesting a specific drug could sway the doctor into the wrong treatment, *most of the time!* So here's an even better reason not to ask for advertised drugs (or any drug for that matter): you are more likely to get treated with an expensive drug you don't need.

Marketed drugs are always patented, costlier products. Unless it is a one-of-a-kind, breakthrough treatment, there are likely to be several treatment choices that are much cheaper. Why ask for the sleeping pill with the butterfly mascot—at over $5.00 per dose—when your doctor can easily choose from a host of others at one-tenth the price?

New *and* Improved?

In 2003 Ely Lilly ran an aggressive direct-to-consumer advertising campaign for their newly approved product, Strattera, a treatment for attention deficit hyperactivity disorder (ADHD). As a result, thousands of adults and parents of affected children went to their doctors clamoring to get it. But when Strattera was tested against other medications used to treat ADHD, there was no convincing evidence it was as effective or well tolerated as traditional treatments.[8] The average retail price for a three-month supply of Strattera at the lowest usual starting dose is $430. Why would you ask your doctor for an expensive, second-rate treatment?

Of course, marketers are always going to insinuate that their product is new and improved over prior treatments, but there may be no proof of any advantage. Remember, drug companies only need to show that a new drug is better than nothing to get it approved.

Don't Play Doctor

Recommending your own treatment grants you a quick MD degree: *Meddlesome Doctor*. Such suggestions steer your doctor away from the effective treatments he has used for years. It takes him out of his game, inviting him to prescribe a treatment with side effects and drug interactions that are less well known to him. I might ask, "With what justification are you making your own treatment recommendations, anyway?

With the medical expertise you gained watching a TV commercial?" If an ad leads you to believe treatment can help, discuss it with your doctor, but do not presume your diagnosis. Convey your symptoms and your desire for help. The only specific request you should make is that any possible treatment be safe, effective, proven, and *affordable*. After that, leave the specific choice of medication to the doctor.

Don't Play Guinea Pig

The lack of experience with new advertised products makes them riskier than time-tested therapies. New drugs are brought to market faster than ever before. The final phase of testing is now done on the public (you), with serious side effects perhaps only discovered later, after they have been on the market for a while.

In March 2002, the Novartis company launched an advertising campaign for their new drug Elidel (pimecrolimus), a prescription cream for the treatment of eczema in adults and children. In addition to television advertising and direct-response TV, they produced print ads, web and email promotions, patient "education" materials, and direct-mail campaigns to consumers. Two years later, Elidel was firmly established as the leading steroid-free eczema treatment. During that time, reports of cancer, including skin malignancies and lymphoma, in adults *and children* treated with Elidel began to accumulate. Ultimately, three years after the drug's introduction, the FDA issued a public health advisory warning about the risk of cancer with topical use of Elidel. Those who succumbed to the allure of the advertising and rushed to get the latest treatment became test cases for the long-term effects. Some ended up trading temporary relief from a benign skin condition for a life-threatening malignancy. How many, had they known the risks, would have opted for safer treatment?

When medication is warranted, you should ask for a drug with a safe and well-established treatment record. If the best possible medication choice happens to be an advertised drug, then that's fine; but your doctor will be making the choice from a position of medical knowledge and experience, and (hopefully) not based on the marketing influence of an advertising campaign.

It Must Be True—I Saw It on TV

Do you believe everything you hear? Of course not! What makes you think drug advertising is held to a higher standard than any other product ballyhoo? The vigilant supervision of the FDA? The unfortunate truth is that the frenzy of prescription drug marketing in recent years has been accompanied by a reduction in oversight by the FDA. Since 2002, citations to drug companies for advertising violations have been delayed in the FDA counsel's office so that (according to a General Accounting Office report), " . . . regulatory letters may not be issued until after the advertising campaign has run its course." The report goes on to say, "FDA's oversight has not prevented some pharmaceutical companies from repeatedly disseminating new misleading advertisements."[9]

But you don't need the FDA to know that drug ads are deceptive. If they boldly proclaim that a new sleeping pill is APPROVED FOR LONG-TERM USE, but later quickly mumble that sleep medicines may lose effectiveness, carry a risk of dependency, and should not be used for extended periods, you *know* it's misleading!

Which Came First—the Diagnosis or the Treatment?

Another problem with prescription drug advertising is that it focuses patients on a treatment rather than on the diagnosis. You may be led to believe that you have the problem the drug treats but actually have something entirely different going on. With incomplete knowledge, patients become convinced of an inaccurate diagnosis and then solicit an inappropriate treatment from the doctor. The rushed physician may be persuaded by patients' enthusiasm for a trial of an advertised drug, take the quick way out of the visit, and give in to their demands with a new prescription for the product. This is what I call LMC: lousy medical care.

Do your pocketbook and your health a favor: do not ask for advertised drugs as a new treatment. If an advertisement motivates you to make an appointment to discuss symptoms, then it *has* done a public service. Just don't presume your diagnosis or request the advertised product for treatment.

Media Mania

Avoid requesting drugs mentioned in news reports of the latest breakthrough treatments. These are often thinly veiled advertisements or press releases originating from the drug companies themselves. Even when the report is on an intriguing new study published in a prestigious medical journal, it is

best to maintain an air of skepticism. Far too often these studies are sponsored by the parent drug company. Even worse,
authors of these studies sometimes have direct financial ties
to the companies whose drugs they are testing. It is disturbing
how often the data is "spun" rather than objectively reported,
and it is deceitful that unfavorable data is sometimes not even
reported at all. As recently as December 2005, none other
than the *New England Journal of Medicine* disclosed that (previously unknown to them) critical data had been withheld from
a study they published on the drug Vioxx in November 2000.[10]
The exclusion resulted in an underestimation of the risk of
heart attack in patients taking the drug.

Celebrities are paid handsomely to promote drugs they
claim have helped them. You may recall Mickey Mantle making the TV talk-show circuit with testimonials of how the drug
Voltaren had helped his arthritis. And who can forget the
novelty of seeing Senator Bob Dole proudly endorsing the
attributes of Viagra? (How embarrassing!) Whether presented
during a commercial break or during the regular program-
ming, it's all advertising and should be viewed critically as
such.

So how can you sort it all out? Well, the axiom *caveat emptor*
("let the buyer beware") continues to provide wisdom today.
Knowledge is power, and I encourage patients to study their
medical conditions and treatments specifically, and health
maintenance and disease prevention in general. Use reliable
sources, such as nonprofit disease foundations (although
these too can be fronts for drug marketing!), academic medi-

cal centers, medical specialty associations, and the National Institutes of Health. Beware of "educational material" originating from commercial interests; this is almost always biased. Most important, though, you need a personal doctor whom you can trust—one who maintains specialty board certification and stays current in medical education and practice. It is primarily the physician's responsibility to keep up with new discoveries within the specialty. There is nothing wrong with discussing how new treatments and studies might affect your management, but trust your doctor to make appropriate treatment recommendations. Just make sure that cost of therapy is one of the considerations.

Take It to the Bank

- Asking for prescription drugs makes it more likely for you to receive them whether needed or not.
- Advertised drugs are expensive patented products that are likely to be a poor value.
- Drug advertising is exaggerated and often misleading.
- Advertised drugs may be riskier and less effective than other available treatments.
- Asking for a specific treatment presumes a diagnosis that may not be correct and increases your chances of receiving an unnecessary treatment.
- Encourage your doctor to help you find the most cost-effective treatments by emphasizing budgetary constraints and avoiding expensive advertised drugs.

CSM 9: "No Thanks, Doc. Keep the Samples"

So, your doctor advises beginning a new long-term treatment with medication. He grabs some colorful boxes out of the cabinet and starts explaining that these free medication samples will give you an opportunity to "try before you buy." Which of the following choices is your best response to bring about the most cost-effective treatment?

A. Listen intently and write down the dosing instructions.
B. Inquire about possible side effects.
C. Ask about dosing in relation to meals.
D. Calmly state, "No thank you, doctor. Keep the samples. Just give me a prescription for a trusted medication that's within my budget."

When the response in that situation routinely becomes "D," we will have begun to return the practice of medicine from a marketing ploy to a science.

What gives? Why not start a new treatment with drug company samples? At least you are sure you got the correct medicine, right? The doctor gave it to you himself. And they're *free!* There is something reassuring in getting a new medication directly from the doctor. You talk over the treatment in the actual presence of the mysterious new pills. It's as if he's saying, "Here it is; this is the best medicine for you." Ah, but is it?

Those sample boxes contain the latest offerings of the pharmaceutical companies. They are almost always under patent (not available as a generic), and they are always among the most expensive prescription drugs. They are much more likely to represent yet another addition to an established class of medication (the overpriced redundant drugs) than to be some new breakthrough drug. Your doctor does not have samples of every available drug. He only has the ones the drug companies would like him to prescribe—the ones that give them the biggest profit. If you could only start treatment with office samples, that would leave out over 99 percent of the possible choices, including the most well-established and proven medicines. Is that good practice? You might well ask your doctor why he is choosing that particular drug to begin with. If it is simply because he has samples, then read him choice "D" above: "No thanks, doc. Just give me the ol' tried-and-true."

Expensive *and* Risky

But don't the doctor's free samples represent the latest, most technologically advanced treatment for your condition? Other than expense, why wouldn't you want something new and improved over some old generic formulation? Keep in mind that your representatives in the US Congress have made it easier and faster than ever before for new drugs to be brought to market. The Prescription Drug User Fee Act of 1992 now allows drug companies to pay fees to speed up drug review time; the required testing and scrutiny of new drugs is not nearly as long or involved as it used to be. Consequently, we are discovering some serious side effects of new medications only after these products have come to market. In October 2006, the *Los Angeles Times* reported that a blue-ribbon panel of the Institute of Medicine* found that the FDA fails to devote

---

* The part of the National Academies that advises the government on scientific and technical issues.

enough energy and resources to monitoring drugs once they are approved. A trusting American public completes the final phase of clinical testing of these new drugs; in essence, you have become a lab rat.

The drug Vioxx is a recent example. Vioxx belonged to a new class of anti-inflammatory drugs called COX-2 inhibitors. With its approval in May 1999, it was touted as being a safer, more effective treatment for arthritic conditions and was marketed heavily to physicians and the public. Doctors, including myself, were starting patients out with stacks of free Vioxx sample boxes provided by friendly sales representatives. More than a million Americans were treated with the drug. Then the long-term data began to accumulate, showing a two-and-a-half times greater probability of stroke and heart attack in steady users of Vioxx. The parent company, Merck, voluntarily pulled the drug from the market in November 2004. As of September 2006, the number of Vioxx-related lawsuits filed against Merck had exceeded 22,000.

The drugs Baycol, Seldane, Posicor, Hismanol, Duract, Propulcid, Raxar, and Lotronex were each withdrawn from the market between 1998 and 2001 after causing fatalities.[11] All had been generously given as samples to physician offices with much fanfare upon initial approval.

In addition to acting quicker to get drugs on the market, the FDA has also been slower to remove new drugs when serious side effects are discovered. Baycol, a cholesterol-lowering drug from the "statin" family, was not withdrawn until August 2001, even though independent case reports and internal company documents revealed an increased risk of muscle-cell destruction called *rhabdomyolosis* in late 1999.[12] When Baycol was used in combination with another cholesterol drug, gemfibrozil, one out of every eleven patients treated for a year could be expected to develop this dangerous side effect.[13] The diabetes drug Rezulin (troglitazone) provides an even more sobering example. Although discontinued in Europe in December 1997, it was not pulled from the US market until March 2000, after sixty-three Americans had died from liver failure as a consequence of taking it.[14]

As of this writing, the arthritis drug Celebrex is still available and widely prescribed even though its use has demonstrated an increased risk of heart attack, stroke, and cardiovascular death. In a study published in the *New England Journal of Medicine* in March 2005, the incidence of cardiovascular disease was 2.4 to 3.3 times higher among two thousand patients taking varying doses of Celebrex, compared to those taking placebos over a three-year period.[15] (In fairness, some of the doses of Celebrex used in the study were higher than those ordinarily used.)

Never mind the cost of these new drugs—with the current system of FDA approval, monitoring, and withdrawal, you may consider it *too risky* to accept treatment with sampled medications! After reviewing much of the data on COX-2 inhibitors, doctors Bruce Soloway and Allan S. Brett, editors of *Journal Watch*, concluded: "Many patients who used COX-2 inhibitors [like Vioxx] could have derived similar benefit from less-expensive agents whose risks were better understood."[16] Wouldn't most patients be better served taking cheaper, well-established medications with known long-term consequences?

Don't be too anxious to try the latest-approved drug for a condition that has a solid treatment record with older agents. The experience of use, and the understanding of the benefits and risks of these agents, make them a safer bet, both for your health and your bank account.

The Great Giveaway

Doctors love to give away free samples. We do it by the bagful. It feels so generous, and the patients seem so appreciative. Filling up a shopping bag with all those neat little boxes of $3-a-pill medicines makes one feel so expansive, like ol' St. Nick himself. However, there is nothing saintly about starting a patient on an expensive patented drug when a cheaper generic medication would do as well or better. The samples eventually run out and, with Christmas over, the patient stands in shock at the pharmacy checkout wondering how he is going to pay for the stuff. Of course, if the best and first choice of new treatment happens to be a new, patented, brand-name medicine, your doctor will surely explain that there are no equivalent alternatives. You must then question her about cost and begin a discussion of how that will fit into your medication budget. In most cases, though, the first choice of treatment will not be in the sample cupboard, and the freebees will actually represent an expensive and risky second-best.

Starting a drug with free samples can also be troublesome to insured patients with prescription drug coverage utilizing a formulary. (A formulary is a list of preferred drugs covered by an insurance or drug-benefit plan.) If the new sample drug is not on the formulary, it will not be covered without special authorization from the insurance company that may be arduous to get. Newer patented drugs that are on the list are likely to require higher co-payments. If you have a drug-benefit plan, always bring a copy of the most recent formulary to your doctor's appointments and check that all new prescriptions are on the formulary before accepting any free samples.

Take It to the Bank

- For initiation of long-term drug treatment, do not accept drug company samples from your doctor.
- Instead, politely say, "No thank you, doctor. Keep the samples. Just give me a prescription for a trusted medicine within my budget."

CSM 10: Insist on Generic Drugs

If medications are going to be a necessary part of your therapy, then pay attention right here because no other cost-saving method saves you as much as using generic drugs. As you can see in table 5-1 (pages 94–95), buying the generic version of the cholesterol drug Zocor (simvastatin) can save over $330 every three months. Ninety generic Prozac (fluoxetine) capsules are $407 cheaper than brand-name. A three-month supply of generic Zantac (ranitidine) is under $25—95 percent less than the brand-name price. So why aren't you getting generics?

Most patients understand that generic drugs are cheaper, but many are uncertain about using them. Will they work as well as the name brand? Who manufactures them? Why are they so cheap? What exactly *is* a generic drug?

What's in a Name?

Pharmaceutical companies coin "brand names" for each of their patented drugs. Lipitor, Prozac, and Viagra are some famous examples. Would you recognize them by their generic names?* The generic name is a standard name that belongs only to the drug and not to any particular company. Generic drugs, then, are copies of brand-name medications made by other manufacturers after the patents expire.

Generic drug makers (Geneva, Mylan, Warrick, to name a few) usually don't develop and test new medicines. They simply manufacture and distribute standard medications that are no longer under patent. They also don't have the obscene marketing and administration budgets of the major pharmaceutical companies. This allows them to price medicines much cheaper than the original brand-name versions. Competition among several manufacturers also helps keep prices low.

Consider the cholesterol-lowering medicine lovastatin, one of three "statin" drugs currently available as a generic. It has been off patent since June 2001. Multiple manufacturers now make it, and the price has come down considerably. The discount Internet price for a ninety-day supply of generic 20 mg lovastatin is $60, or 67 cents a pill. Using table 5-6, compare that to Lipitor's discount Internet price. Ninety of the 20 mg pills cost $336, or $3.73 per pill—over five and a half times as much!

---

* Answer: atorvastatin, fluoxetine, and sildenafil, respectively.

Even though a drug patent has expired, the brand name still belongs to the original company. Other companies may then designate their own brand names for the same drug or sell it with the generic name. The blood pressure drug diltiazem, for example, was originally patented under the name Cardizem by Hoechst, Marion, Roussel, Inc. (now Aventis Pharmaceuticals). After the patent expired, various other manufacturers patented their own brand names for extended-release forms of the drug. So if your doctor writes the generic name "diltiazem, extended release" on your prescription, you may receive a bottle with Cardizem CD, Cartia XT, Dilacor, Diltia XT, Taztia, Tiamate, or Tiazac written on the label. The tablets or capsules each have a distinctive appearance unique to the manufacturer, but they are all still just good ol' diltiazem. No wonder you're confused!

If your doctor writes a brand name for a particular medication on your prescription and includes the letters DAW ("dispense as written") or DNS ("do not substitute"),* the pharmacist cannot substitute a generic equivalent. Without this designation, the pharmacist may substitute a generic equivalent. In this case the tablets or capsules may look different from refill to refill. Pharmaceutical companies encourage doctors to specify their brand with the DAW or DNS written on the prescription. But if you want the best possible price for a medicine that is no longer patented, make sure that these designations are omitted. That way the pharmacist can give you the cheapest option from among available formulations.

---

* Or similar designations, depending on the state in which you live.

A Rose Is a Rose

But will a generically manufactured medicine be as effective as the originally patented brand name? The FDA requires that generic drugs be manufactured to strict specifications. The chemical structure of the active ingredient must be identical to that of the original "pioneer" drug. The milligram strength must also be precise, so that dosages are equivalent. However, how the medicine is packaged into a tablet or capsule can effect how it is absorbed into the body. The extent that a medicine is assimilated into the body and becomes active is called *bioavailability.*

The FDA requires that generic drugs have a bioavailability no more than 25 percent higher or 20 percent lower than the original product. In practicality, measured bioavailability values for generic drugs are typically within 3 percent of the brand-name original. According to the *Medical Letter on Drugs and Therapeutics*, no well-documented therapeutic differences between brand-name and FDA-approved generics have been reported.[17] Of course, results are what count in the final analysis. If your blood pressure is still well controlled with the new generic batch of pills, then any possible difference in bioavailability is unimportant. Is your cholesterol still controlled on generic zocor? Then don't worry about bioavailability. If, however, you do not see the same effectiveness after switching to a generic drug, an adjustment in the dosage may be all that is required to equalize the effect.

Table 5-1 lists several of the most widely prescribed drugs available in both brand-name and generic forms. The cost for three month's supply of each at the typical lowest starting dose is listed with actual and percentage savings. As you can see, the savings are substantial, sometimes more than 90 percent.

TABLE 5-1: Price Comparison of Some Brand-Name Drugs and Their Generic Equivalents				
Brand-name drug	Price *	Generic equivalent	Price *	Savings (%)
Ambien 10 mg	$391	zolpedem 10 mg	$42	$349 (89%)
Ativan 0.5 mg	$135	lorazepam 0.5 mg	$34	$101 (75%)
Celexa 40 mg	$292	citalopram 40 mg	$75	$217 (74%)
Glucophage 1 g**	$358	metformin 1000 mg	$86	$272 (76%)
Glucotrol 10 mg**	$188	glipizide 10 mg	$22	$166 (88%)
Lopid 600 mg**	$389	gemfibrozil 600 mg	$46	$343 (88%)
Neurontin 800 mg	$363	gabapentin 800 mg	$73	$290 (80%)
Prilosec 20 mg	$406	omeprazole 20 mg	$64	$342 (84%)
Prozac 20 mg	$434	fluoxetine 20 mg	$27	$407 (94%)
Soma 350 mg	$417	carisopridol 350 mg	$32	$385 (92%)
Vicodin ES	$119	hydrocodone/ APAP 7.5/500 mg	$23	$96 (81%)

 * Discount Internet price for a ninety-day supply.
** Dosed twice a day.

(continues on page 96)

TABLE 5-1: Price Comparison of Some Brand-Name Drugs and Their Generic Equivalents, *continued*				
Brand-name drug	**Price ***	**Generic equivalent**	**Price ***	**Savings (%)**
Xanax 0.5 mg	$143	alprazolam 0.5 mg	$11	$132 (92%)
Zantac 300 mg	$460	ranitidine 300 mg	$25	$435 (95%)
Zestril 10 mg	$130	lisinopril 10 mg	$32	$98 (75%)
Zocor 20 mg	$405	simvastatin 20 mg	$74	$331 (82%)
Zoloft 50 mg	$256	sertraline 50 mg	$21	$235 (92%)

* Discount Internet price for a ninety-day supply.

When a Rose Is Not a Rose

Of course, there are exceptions. A very few drugs have what is called a "narrow therapeutic index." This means that the range between too low and too high of a dose is small. Due to slight differences in bioavailability, changes from brand to brand, brand to generic, or from one generic to another can result in over- or undertreatment. The most commonly prescribed medication with a narrow therapeutic index is the thyroid hormone levothyroxine (brand names Levothroid, Levoxyl, and Synthroid). Switching among the brands or to any of several generics could result in symptoms of an under- or overactive thyroid gland. In general, for these drugs it is best to stick with a single manufacturer. Most brands and generics go for about 20¢ –30¢ a pill, so it doesn't matter much which one you get. (The cost is slightly higher for the Levoxyl and Synthroid brands.) Just don't switch products with subsequent prescriptions. If you are taking a proprietary version of levothyroxine, have your doctor write the brand name and "DAW" or "DNS" on the prescription. If you must switch manufacturers, be sure to have your doctor order a thyroid blood test (TSH) four to six weeks afterward to monitor the change.

Drugs with a narrow therapeutic index are listed in table 5-2. As with levothyroxine, you should not change from any of these to a different brand name or generic without physician supervision. For any of these drugs, blood tests may be used to monitor changes in therapy.

TABLE 5-2: Drugs with a Narrow Therapeutic Index
Antiseizure medications
Depakene (valproic acid), Depakote (divalproex), Dilantin (phenytoin), Tegretol (carbamazepine)
Asthma medications
TheoDur/Theo-24 (theophylline)
Blood thinners
Coumadin (warfarin)
Heart medications
Digitek/Lanoxin (digoxin)
Psychiatric medications
Eskalith/Lithobid (lithium)

Expensive-Drug Survival Index

Many popular drugs are listed in the Expensive-Drug Survival Index of this book. Those with an available generic are indicated by a "G" in the first column. For maximum economy, always insist on generic formulations of these medications.

Beware of Medicines with a CD, CR, ER, LA, SR, XL, XR, or XT

This advice could be a cost-saving method all by itself. When you see these symbols added to the name of your medicine (meant to indicate "continuous delivery," "extended-release," and the like), think "extended profit." The major pharmaceutical companies make their profits on the sale of their patented brand-name drugs. When a patent expires, only a fraction of sales for the drug will stay with the company as people switch to cheaper generics. Sales of a blockbuster drug can plunge 80 percent or more the first year after a generic competitor hits the market.[18] Facing these revenue losses, company executives will do whatever they can to milk the profits of their previously exclusive cash cow.

One scheme to keep the flow of prescription dollars in the company has been to repackage the same old product with a new patent. Drug companies come out with extended-release formulations before the patent on the original drug expires. The drug has not been changed, but the way the medicine is absorbed or released into the body is altered. These "new" drugs have their own patents extending out far beyond the expiration of the original drug's patent. This scheme is in effect a back-door extension of the patent. Company executives know that patients switched to the new extended-release version will not be lost to generic competitors later, and with aggressive marketing an extended-release product helps keep sales profits at home.

Paxil CR

Consider the patented antidepressant Paxil CR. In this case the CR stands for "controlled release." The manufacturer, GlaxoSmithKline, states that Paxil CR has the advantage of a Geomatrix tablet that delays absorption of the drug, releasing it gradually into the system rather than all at once. Sounds good in theory, but the duration of action of regular Paxil is already so long as to allow convenient once-a-day dosing. Moreover, there have been no controlled studies to prove any advantage of Paxil CR over regular Paxil. When Paxil was first introduced in 1993 it was, of course, the only form of paroxitine available. It was a highly effective treatment for depression and anxiety disorders and was soon grossing GlaxoSmithKline billions of dollars per year in sales. That's a lot of revenue to lose to the generic wolves waiting for the patent to expire. Hence, Paxil CR emerged before Paxil was scheduled to lose its patent. Patients prescribed this new formulation do not have the option for the cheaper generic version. As long as the doctor writes "CR" on the prescription, only the brand-name product can be dispensed by the pharmacist.

Wellbutrin SR and Wellbutrin XL

Some companies have used this same scheme more than once with the same drug! The antidepressant Wellbutrin (bupropion) was first approved in 1985. Its shorter duration of action necessitated three-times-a-day dosing. Wellbutrin SR (offering twice-a-day dosing) came out in October 1996, thirty-eight months before original Wellbutrin went generic. Then, in August 2003, Wellbutrin XL (dosed once a day) was introduced, just five months before the SR version went off patent. Granted, although immediate release bupropion is less convenient at three doses a day than twice a day for the SR version and once daily for the XL, the cost variation is considerable. The average retail price for a three-month supply of generic bupropion (at 300 mg a day in divided doses) is $270, while Wellbutrin SR and Wellbutrin XL at the same daily dose are $693 and $656 respectively. For the best combination of convenience and price, savvy consumers should insist on the *generic* SR formulation, available for the discount Internet price of $164 for a three-month supply.

We Have a Winner: Cardizem SR, Cardizem CD, and Cardizem LA!

No drug company has used the extended-release game to protect their profits more than Aventis Pharmaceuticals with their blockbuster blood pressure drug Cardizem. Not since *Wheel of Fortune* has adding letters been so profitable! Cardizem was approved in November 1982. The SR version came out in 1989, the CD version in 1991, and the LA version in 2003. Each new approval has enabled the marketing of the familiar Cardizem brand name to continue for more than two decades. All of these formulations contain the same calcium channel blocker diltiazem. Doctors and patients seem more than happy to stick by it, even though generic extended-release diltiazem has been available since 1993 at a much cheaper price. The LA and CD versions both offer once-a-day dosing but cost up to twice as much as the generic once-a-day diltiazem ER.

Toprol-XL

Metoprolol is a beta-adrenergic receptor antagonist (beta-blocker) used for the treatment of high blood pressure, angina, arrhythmias, and congestive heart failure. In 1992, the extended-release formulation of metoprolol, Toprol-XL, was approved by the FDA. In direct comparison trials, Toprol-XL administered once a day was as effective as immediate-release metoprolol dosed one or more times a day. In the prescribing information for Toprol-XL, the company uses data on the effectiveness of immediate-release metoprolol to justify the use of the extended-release Toprol-XL.

Granted, once-a-day dosing is more convenient, but it's also more expensive. The discount Internet price for a three-month supply of the 100 mg Toprol-XL is about $120, but three months of the same dose of generic metoprolol (taken as 50 mg twice a day) goes for $27 (see table 5-4). That's quite a difference for one less dose per day. In practice, many doctors are prescribing extended-release metoprolol two or more times a day anyway. So why was Toprol-XL the fourteenth-most-often prescribed drug in America in 2004 while generic metoprolol wasn't even in the top thirty? I attribute it to marketing. The parent company, AstraZenica, has done a great job in getting physicians to prescribe its extended-release product. This might be good news for shareholders in AstraZenica, but it's a boondoggle for patients. Certainly, there may be a few instances where only the extended-release Toprol-XL would be appropriate, but for the majority of patients the XL formulation is simply a waste of money.

Exceptions

Of course, there are always exceptions. There are cases where an extended-release medication avoids serious side effects compared to the immediate-release formulation. Short-acting calcium channel blockers such as nifedipine are an example. These drugs are usually prescribed only in the extended-release form to avoid sudden drops in blood pressure.[19] It would not be appropriate to ask your doctor for the immediate-release type as a cost-saving measure. Anyway, the extended-release version of nifedipine is generically available and is reasonably priced.

Introduction of the continuous-release form of carbidopa/levodopa (Sinemet CR) might be considered a breakthrough in treatment for patients with Parkinson's disease. This formulation simplifies the complicated dosing schedules and alleviates the intermittent periods of impaired movement associated with the immediate-release treatment. And like nifedipine, Sinemet CR is now available as a generic.

Case Study
CSM 10: Request Generic Drugs

Eleanor is a seventy-nine-year-old woman with coronary heart disease and high blood pressure. After coronary bypass surgery, she developed an abnormally fast heart rhythm (tachyarrhythmia). Her cardiologist brought her blood pressure and heart rhythm under control with Cardizem CD 180 mg once daily, and Toprol XL 25 mg three times a day. The only problem was that the price tag for a three-month supply of the two drugs was $543.

With the specialist's approval, I switched Eleanor's medications to a generic brand of Cardizem CD and to the immediate-release form of Toprol XL (metoprolol) at the same respective doses. A twenty-four-hour EKG showed no tachyarrhythmia or other abnormalities, and blood pressure remained well controlled. By obtaining generics and avoiding unnecessary use of brand-name extended-release drugs, Eleanor's cost for three months of treatment was reduced to $185.

Yearly Savings: $1,432

Take It to the Bank

- Find out which of your medications are brand-name drugs and which of those have an available generic formulation. The Expensive-Drug Survival Index at the end of this book has a "G" next to brand names with generic availability as of March 2008. Your pharmacist, a pharmacy website, or a drug reference book can also provide this information.
- Unless there are special circumstances (such as with drugs with a narrow therapeutic index), insist on generic substitutions for all current prescriptions.
- Insist that your doctor leave off the designations "DAW," "DNS," or equivalent from all prescriptions, so that cheaper generic medications may always be substituted.
- Ask your doctor to choose medications that have a generic equivalent for all new prescriptions when appropriate.
- Question your doctor about the necessity of taking patented medicines with the letters CD, CR, ER, LA, SR,

XL, XR, or XT attached to the name. These are usually extended- or controlled-release versions of generically available (or soon-to-be-available) immediate-release medications. Often, the only advantage of these drugs is the convenience of less frequent dosing. Some have no practical advantage. All are usually more expensive than their immediate-release generic equivalents.

CSMs 11 and 12 discuss ways to take advantage of generic pricing even if your present prescriptions are only available as expensive brand names.

CSM 11: Insist on Cheaper Medicines within the Same Class

How do physicians maintain practical knowledge of all the thousands of different medications available today—not just the names, but the indications and contraindications, effects and side effects, tablet strengths and dosing intervals, and the possible drug-to-drug interactions? The truth is we don't. Physicians only need to know about general classifications of medicines and then become familiar with a few of the choices within each class.

Although there are more than one hundred medicines for the treatment of high blood pressure, all can be placed into nine classes. (Table 5-3 lists the classes of antihypertension drugs.) When a doctor considers new treatment for a patient with high blood pressure, he will first determine which class is best suited as a treatment and then choose a drug from that class. If it is agreed upon to begin with a beta-blocker, for example, the doctor will choose a favored one with which he has had previous experience and success (or perhaps one he has company samples of in the cabinet). Drugs within a class have similar properties, and some are almost identical, so there is no need to be fluent in the use of every one of them. Most physicians form their own repertoire of favorite medications, routinely prescribing only a few drugs from each class. We develop these habits for a variety of reasons, but cost to the patient is usually *not* one of them!

| **TABLE 5-3: Classes of Drugs for Treatment of High Blood Pressure** ||
Medication class	**Examples***
Alpha-1 blockers (the "azosins")	Cardura (doxazosin), prazosin, Hytrin (terazosin)
Angiotensin-converting enzyme (ACE) inhibitors (the "prils")	Altace (ramipril), lisinopril, Accupril (quinapril)
Angiotensin II receptor blockers (ARBs) (the "sartans")	Avapro (irbesartan), Cozaar (losartan), Diovan (valsartan)
Beta-blockers (the "lols")	atenolol, propranolol, Toprol-XL (metoprolol)
with alpha-1 blocking activity	Coreg (carvedilol), labetalol
Calcium channel blockers	Cardizem, Diltia, and Tiazac (diltiazem), Norvasc (amlodipine), verapamil
Central alpha-2 agonists	clonidine, guanabenz, guanfacine
Direct vasodilators	hydralazine, minoxidil
Diuretics	hydrochlorothiazide, furosemide, spironolactone
Peripheral adrenergic neuron antagonists	guanadrel, reserpine

* Brand-name drugs are capitalized.

When Choices = Bargains

Toprol-XL is a commonly prescribed medication for high blood pressure. It belongs to the class of *beta-adrenergic blocking drugs*, or beta-blockers. Other beta-blockers include Bystolic, Corgard, Inderal, Kerlone, Tenormin, and Zebeta. All have the basic property of blocking specific nerve receptors, ultimately lowering blood pressure, but there are some differences. The duration of action and dosing intervals are different. The milligram strengths are different. *And* prices at the pharmacy are also definitely different!

We can thank competition among the pharmaceutical companies and a business concept called "market share" for the number of choices within each drug class. (And where there are choices, there may be bargains.) When a new drug class is developed and becomes a popular mode of treatment, the first company on the scene reaps the benefit. Other companies soon follow suit and come out with their own additions to the class. Once approved, these new drugs can be aggressively marketed to obtain the biggest possible slice of the sales pie.

Within each drug class, the major pharmaceutical companies develop and market one or more medicines competing for market share. Pricing among drugs in a class varies considerably. Table 5-4 lists cost differences among some brand-name and generic beta-blockers. The cost for three months' therapy ranges from $442 for the most expensive brand-name drug, Inderal LA, to only $12 for generic atenolol.

Knowledge of these pricing differences can save you a lot. Imagine that your doctor recommends starting beta-blocker therapy for high blood pressure and begins writing a prescription for Inderal LA. Even the generic version at the discount Internet price is going to set you back $126 every three months. Wouldn't it be great to know what cheaper drugs from the same class are available? Using the Expensive-Drug Survival Index at the end of this book, and checking prices, you would learn that atenolol is less than one-tenth the cost of generic Inderal LA. You could then ask your doctor why he is choosing the more expensive proprietary drug. Chances are there is no justification, and the cheaper medicine could be tried first, saving you over $450 a year.

Why would pharmaceutical companies price their drugs so much higher than other drugs within the same class? Because they can! All prices have been carefully set by the parent companies to maximize their profits. Whether due to name recognition, physician allegiance, advertising, or some

TABLE 5-4: Some Beta-Blockers		
Brand name (generic name)	Brand-name price*	Generic price*
Bystolic (nebivolol) 5 mg	$156	N/A
Corgard (nadolol) 20 mg	$186	$22
Inderal (propranolol) 10 mg**	$80	$16
Inderal LA (propranolol) 120 mg	$442	$126
Kerlone (betaxolol) 10 mg	$121	$90
Lopressor (metoprolol) 50 mg**	$250	$27
Tenormin (atenolol) 25 mg	$141	$12
Toprol-XL (metoprolol) 100 mg	$120	$100
Zebeta (bisoprolol) 5 mg	$254	$93

  * Discount Internet price for a ninety-day supply.
 ** Dosed twice a day.

other reason, if the drug is selling well, marketing executives will price it to their best advantage. But knowledge of the competition for market share can work to your advantage. There are excellent medications in every drug class that sell at substantially cheaper prices than the others.

Consider the class of high blood pressure drugs called *angiotensin-converting enzyme inhibitors* (ACE inhibitors). As you can see in table 5-5, brand-name Vasotec sells for $230 for ninety days' treatment. Altace goes for $166. Generic lisinopril is a bargain at $32 for three months' supply, and generic captopril beats all at $23. From $230 to $23 is quite a variation among drugs that all work in the same way. Surely most people

TABLE 5-5: Some Angiotensin-Converting Enzyme (ACE) Inhibitors		
Brand name (generic name)	**Brand-name price***	**Generic price***
Accupril (quinapril) 5 mg	$142	$51
Aceon (perindopril) 2 mg	$142	Available soon
Altace (ramipril) 2.5 mg	$166	$136
Capoten (captopril) 12.5 mg**	No longer available	$23
Lotensin (benazepril) 10 mg	$132	$65
Mavik (trandolapril) 2 mg	$119	$100
Monopril (fosinopril) 10 mg	$129	$90
Prinivil (lisinopril) 10 mg	$96	$32
Univasc (moexipril) 7.5 mg	$120	Available soon
Vasotec (enalapril) 2.5 mg**	$230	$34
Zestril (lisinopril) 10 mg	$130	$32

* Discount Internet price for a ninety-day supply.
** Dosed twice a day.

are prescribed the generic captopril for the best economy of treatment, right? Not so—in 2005 four times as many prescriptions were written for Altace as for captopril, at over seven times the cost! Twice as many prescriptions were filled for quinapril, at double the price.* That's a lot of unnecessarily expensive prescriptions. If only the folks taking these drugs could discuss cheaper alternatives in the class with their doctors. Perhaps those who are having trouble affording medicines could switch to the more economical captopril, enalapril, or once-a-day lisinopril, at a 60 to 90 percent savings.

Top of the Class?

Sometimes physicians choose a specific drug because of benefits shown in clinical studies. Such has been the case with Altace. The HOPE study, published in the *New England Journal of Medicine* in January 2000, showed that treatment of high-risk patients with Altace reduced the incidence of heart attack, stroke, or cardiovascular death by 22 percent, compared to those treated with a placebo.[20] These clinical trials motivate physicians to choose the specific drug used in the study rather than another from the same class. That helps explains the thirteen million prescriptions for Altace in 2004. Of course it doesn't hurt that the parent companies also cite these studies in sales promotions. ** The HOPE study has not been repeated with all of the ACE inhibitors, so whether that protection extends to the entire class is unproven. And there

  * According to Rxlist.com.
 ** It is also interesting to note that the manufacturers of Altace were the ones who sponsored the HOPE study.

are no large-scale, head-to-head comparison trials to prove clinically relevant differences in these agents.* Any advantage of Altace over other ACE inhibitors for heart attack patients or others at high risk for cardiovascular disease is speculative. Most taking ACE inhibitors will not fall into these categories anyway. So if you have not had a heart attack, or are not at high risk for one, there is really no rationale for using Altace over a cheaper ACE inhibitor.

Class Warfare

Many classes of drugs will have one or more generic choices. At no time will choosing an alternative drug within a given class provide greater savings than when one of the members has gone generic. The statin class, prescribed to lower cholesterol, provides a perfect example. Among the statin drugs, listed in table 5-6, the generic lovastatin, pravastatin, and simvistatin are significantly cheaper than the brand-name drugs. Ninety 20 mg Lipitor tablets sell for $336, but the same amount of pravastatin goes for $45.

Despite the marked discount with generic statins, expensive brand names are prescribed far more frequently. Lipitor and Zocor were among the top twenty-five drugs prescribed in 2005, with over eighty-five million prescriptions written, while lovastatin was not even in the top seventy, with less than one-eighth as many prescriptions.** This is a huge difference—especially when you consider that no head-to-head trials have

* Canadian researchers observed superior risk reduction in heart attack patients treated with Altace compared to other ACE inhibitors, but those patients also got more beta-blockers and statins.[21]

** Rxlist.com.

directly shown these popular brand-name drugs to be any better at preventing vascular disease than lovastatin.

But is it reasonable to just switch medications within the same class and expect the same results? Remember, to get FDA approval, drug companies only need to show that their product is more effective than a placebo, that is, that it's better than nothing. Surprisingly few studies comparing drugs of the same class are published, or if they are, the methods may be questionable. Pfizer, the manufacturer of Lipitor, sponsored a clinical trial comparing their drug to Pravachol in reducing coronary artery plaques (the REVERSAL study). Whereas there was no plaque progression in the patients who took Lipitor (compared to a 3 percent increase with Pravachol), those patients received 80 mg per day, while the patients receiving Pravachol got only 40 mg.[22] Knowing Lipitor to be more potent anyway, how is that comparison going to help decide which drug might be better?

TABLE 5-6: Some Cholesterol-Lowering Drugs		
Brand name (generic name)	**Brand-name price***	**Generic price* (or patent expiration date)**
Altoprev (lovastatin) 20 mg	$361	(2017)
Crestor (rosuvastatin) 20 mg	$296	(2016)
Lescol (fluvastatin) 20 mg	$230	(2012)
Lescol XL (fluvastatin) 80 mg	$292	(2012)
Lipitor (atorvastatin) 20 mg	$336	(2009)
Mevacor (lovastatin) 20 mg	$200	$60
Pravachol (pravastatin) 20 mg	$290	$45
Zocor (simvastatin) 20 mg	$405	$74

* Discount Internet price for a ninety-day supply.

They did it again in the IDEAL Study, pitting high-dose Lipitor against "usual-dose" Zocor. I'm not an expert in clinical research, but that seems like two different variables to me. Either compare high-dose Lipitor to usual-dose Lipitor, or compare Lipitor to Zocor at the same dose, but not both at the same time. It's no surprise that this study was also sponsored by Pfizer and that five of the authors disclosed financial ties to the company.[23]

Without better comparison trials, it will be unclear how switching drugs within a class may affect your treatment. A cheaper alternative may work a little better or worse. Dosage adjustments may make any real differences in effectiveness inconsequential. If your cholesterol is still as low with lovastatin as it was on Lipitor, it may be well worth the switch. One thing is certain, though: lovastatin at any dose works better than a prescription of Lipitor that is never purchased because it is too expensive.

A Change for the Cheaper

But surely there are some medical conditions for which medications should not be changed just to save a few bucks, right? Let me say now—no effective therapy for *any* medical condition should be changed without absolute indication. One of the most valuable lessons of my training was stated succinctly (if not in the best English) by my mentor Dr. Michael Caruso, who said, "If it ain't broke, don't fix it." However, these methods are suggested in response to a system of medicine in this country that is "broke" for many people. Changing medications for financial reasons is justified if you cannot reasonably afford your present treatment.

Table 5-7 lists the antidepressants known as selective serotonin reuptake inhibitors (SSRIs). Cost of three months' therapy with these drugs ranges from as high as $434 to as low as $21. But shouldn't the choice among these important medications be highly individualized regardless of cost? Well, according to the *Medical Letter on Drugs and Therapeutics*, "There is no good evidence that any SSRI is superior to any other for treatment of depression or any other indication for which these drugs are used. Since all SSRIs in adequate doses are about equally [effective], the choice among them comes down to adverse effects, drug interactions, and cost."[24]

So unless you know of any drug interactions or adverse effects, it would make most sense from an economical standpoint to begin drug therapy for depression with an inexpensive SSRI, such as fluoxetine. Nevertheless, doctors prescribed Zoloft, Lexapro, and Celexa—at eight times the price—over sixty million times in 2004, three times as often as fluoxetine.

TABLE 5-7: Some Drugs for Depression (SSRIs)		
Brand name (generic name)	Brand-name price*	Generic price* (or patent expiration date)
Celexa (citalopram) 20 mg	$280	$90
Lexapro (escitalopram) 10 mg	$229	(2012)
Paxil (paroxitine) 20 mg	$288	$29
Paxil CR (paroxitine) 25 mg	$298	Available soon
Prozac (fluoxetine) 20 mg	$434	$27
Prozac Weekly (fluoxetine) 90 mg**	$310	(2017)
Zoloft (sertraline) 50 mg	$256	$21

* Discount Internet price for a ninety-day supply.
** Dosed once a week.

If you are doing well on one of the more expensive drugs, I would not encourage you to change medicines. However, if you cannot afford the treatment, or have stopped taking it due to cost, a change to one of the cheaper SSRIs might be reasonable.

Expensive-Drug Survival Index

I would not expect most physicians to know the relative prices of all the drugs in a particular class. But there is no reason that *you* cannot find out the best values and take the information to your doctor. The most popular expensive drugs are listed alphabetically in the Expensive-Drug Survival Index of this book. If cheaper medications from the same class are available, they are listed in the "Same-class substitutions" column to the right. At your treatment review visit, ask your doctor if one of these or another inexpensive medicine from the same class could be substituted as a cost-saving measure. If possible, shop ahead of time and be ready to show your doctor how much you would save with the change.

> Say you are well treated with Nexium for heartburn, but the $547 per quarter ransom makes it painful to swallow. Checking the Expensive-Drug Survival Index, we find that Nexium has a same-family substitution, omeprazole. A quick price check on DestinationRx.com shows that Costco sells 90 capsules of omeprazole for just $66. You could then bring these price comparisons to your doctor to discuss (demand?) a possible substitution. A $1,900 per year spoonful of savings sure helps the medicine go down!

Of course not every costly medicine will have a cheaper cousin. If not, the same-class substitution column in the survival index will be blank. The good news is that if your expensive drug is in the index at all, one or another of cost-saving methods 10–13 will apply. If your drug is not listed in the index, perhaps one of the other CSMs will help. Still, for any expensive drug, it never hurts to ask your doctor, "Is there a cheaper substitution from the same class that I could take instead?"

Case Study
CSM 11: Insist on Cheaper Medicines within the Same Class

J.D. is a seventy-four-year-old retired water-well driller who was diagnosed with precancerous changes of the swallowing tube, called Barrett's esophagus. His gastroenterologist prescribed long-term treatment with the acid-blocking drug Protonix, one of the class of medicines called *proton pump inhibitors* (PPIs). In June 2006 J.D. reported to me that the cost of Protonix at our local drugstore was about $3.50 *per tablet*. This seemed outrageous to us both, so I recommended he try switching to another drug from the family of PPIs, the generically available omeprazole.* J.D. found he could buy omeprazole locally for about $1.00 a pill, a 70 percent savings.

Yearly Savings: $913

---

* Omeprazole is the cheapest in the PPI family. It is also available without a prescription. Anyone taking an expensive PPI should discuss the suitability of changing to omeprazole with his or her doctor.

Take It to the Bank

- There are often several drug choices within a particular class, and some are cheaper than others.
- Check the Expensive-Drug Survival Index for each of your costly medicines and note any "same-class substitutions."
- Compare prices of these drugs with the price of your present treatment online or at your pharmacy.
- Ask your doctor if a substitution is appropriate, and show her the potential savings.
- To keep treatment affordable, always insist that your doctor prescribe cheaper drugs within a medication class.

CSM 12: Insist on a Cheaper Class for the Same Treatment Goal

CSM 11 showed us how different medicines in the same class can differ substantially in price, especially if one or more has gone generic. It is also true that different classes used to treat the same condition can show significant cost variation. If all the medications within a particular class are unsuitable or beyond your budget, then perhaps a drug from a different class can do the job.

Hay Fever Hysteria

Flonase is a heavily marketed and commonly prescribed steroid nasal spray for the treatment of allergies. Doctors wrote fifteen million prescriptions for Flonase in 2005. The discount Internet price for a ninety-day supply is about $250. The other brand-name nasal steroid sprays—Nasonex, Nasacort AQ, and Rhinocort Aqua—go for about the same. Seventeen million prescriptions were written for these three allergy medicines in 2005. That seems like a lot of money going up the nose of America to help keep allergy symptoms under control. Isn't there a cheaper class of drugs to treat allergies?

Classes of medicine for treatment of nasal allergies are listed in table 5-8. The cheapest allergy medicines belong to the nonprescription antihistamine class. A single 4 mg tablet of the antihistamine chlopheniramine (Clor-Tri-Meton and others) offers allergy sufferers up to six hours of relief for less than ten cents. A three-month supply of once-a-day, nonsedating loratadine (Alavert, Claritin, Tavist ND, and others) costs as little as $25. Benadryl (diphenhydramine) and Tavist (clemastine) are other antihistamines available over the counter (OTC) at just pennies a pill. Antihistamines may not be for every allergy patient; they may cause confusion or loss of balance in the elderly, and they may contribute to prostate symptoms in older men. But I have to wonder how many patients prescribed expensive nasal steroid sprays were ever informed of the option of inexpensive OTC antihistamines.

There is a wide spectrum of pricing among antihistamines, the most expensive being the prescription brands Allegra and Clarinex. These can cost even more than the nasal steroids (even though they have not been shown to be as effective), and they should ideally be reserved for those for whom loratadine or other cheaper antihistamines have failed to work. Nevertheless, thanks to aggressive marketing, doctors prescribed these high-priced drugs (along with the then-patented Zyrtec) almost thirty-four million times in 2005. If you are using any expensive allergy treatment and have not taken OTC antihistamines in a while, ask your doctor about giving them another try. Along with cromolyn sodium nasal spray and decongestants, these economical alternatives could save you hundreds of dollars per year.

TABLE 5-8: Classes of Drugs for Nasal Allergies		
Drug class	**Examples**	**Price***
Corticosteroid nasal sprays	flunisolide (Nasalide, Nasarel)	$106**
	Flonase (fluticasone)	$250
	Nasacort AQ (triamcinolone)	$258
	Nasonex (mometasone)	$250
	Rhinocort Aqua (budesonide)	$259
Antihistamines, available without prescription (OTC)	cetirizine (Zyrtec)	$30**
	chlorpheniramine (Clor-Tri-Meton and others)	$70**
	diphenhydramine (Benadryl and others)	$43**
	loratadine (Alavert, Claritin, Tavist ND)	$26**
	Tavist-1 (clemastine)	$97
Antihistamines, requiring a prescription	Allegra (fexofenadine)	$288
	Clarinex (desloratadine)	$320
Antihistamine/ decongestant combinations (prescription)	Allegra-D (fexofenadine/pseudoephedrine)	$316
	Clarinex-D (desloratidine/pseudoephedrine)	$321
Antihistamine nasal spray	Astellin (azelastine)	$268
Mast cell stablizer	NasalCrom (cromolyn sodium)	$44
Decongestants	pseudoephedrine (Sudafed and others)	$42
Leukotriene blocker	Singulair (montelukast)	$324

  * Discount Internet price for a ninety-day supply.
** Generic price.

The Dirt on Diabetes

The thiazolidinediones (*glitazones*, for short, since nobody can say "thiazolidinediones") represent a newer class of medicine for diabetes. Currently, Actos and Avandia are the only two glitazones available for use in the United States, and both are expensive. These drugs allow the cells of the body to be more sensitive to natural insulin, improving glucose metabolism and thus helping to normalize blood sugar. They began as a welcome addition to our arsenal of medications—the more resources we have to manage diabetes, the better. But when medication is required, if there are several class options, why not take cost (and safety) into consideration?

One of the main goals in the management of diabetes is to normalize blood sugar. Although the mode of action is varied, all of the classes of diabetes medications work toward this goal. There are particular benefits of and drawbacks to each class, of course, but cost may be factored into the choice.

Table 5-9 lists medications used to treat diabetes by class.* Included are the discount Internet prices for ninety days' treatment. As you can see, Actos and Avandia (the glitazones) sell for $506 and $339 for ninety days' treatment. Compare that to metformin, of the biguanide class, or glipizide, of the sulfonurea class, which go for $66 and $15. That kind of difference can really add up! But how do these drugs compare in effectiveness? A study published in the *Journal of Clinical Endocrinology and Metabolism* showed almost identical control

---

* I am not including the older, first generation sulfonureas (e.g., Diabenase, Orinase, and Tolanase) because their use is substandard in the modern treatment of diabetes.

of blood sugar in diabetic patients treated with either metformin or Avandia.[25] Yet, compared to metformin, the cost for
one year's treatment with Avandia is about $1,100 more. Factor
in findings that use of Avandia is associated with an increase
in heart attacks and heart failure, and the better choice of
therapy is clear.[26]

Consider the newest oral drug for diabetes, Januvia. Since
this medication works in a new way compared to other available drugs, it might be considered to be an innovative or
breakthrough drug. Of course, it is always nice to have another

TABLE 5-9: Classes of Drugs for Type II Diabetes		
Drug class	**Examples**	**Price***
Sulfonureas	glimepiride (Amaryl) 2 mg	$19
	glipizide (Glucotrol) 5 mg	$15
	glyburide (Diabeta, Micronase) 2.5 mg	$22
Biguanides	metformin (Glucophage) 500 mg	$66
Thiazolidinediones	Actose (pioglitazone) 30 mg	$506
	Avandia (rosiglitazone) 4 mg	$339
Alpha-glucosidase inhibitors	Precose (acarbose) 25 mg**	$239
	Glyset (miglitol) 25 mg**	$210
Nonsulfonurea insulin secretagogues	Starlix (nateglinide) 120 mg	$398
	Prandin (repaglinide) 0.5 mg	$386
DPP-4 inhibitors	Januvia (sitagliptin) 100 mg	$486
Combinations	Actoplus Met (pioglitazone/metformin) 15 mg/500 mg	$260
	Avandamet (rosaglitazone/metformin) 4 mg/500 mg	$339
	Avandaryl (rosaglitazone/glimepiride) 4 mg/2 mg	$360

  * Discount Internet price for a ninety-day supply.
 ** Dosed three times a day before meals.

choice, but the number of well-established oral medicines available should make Januvia a second-line agent for difficult cases. Clinical trials show Januvia is not as effective in lowering elevated blood sugar as the diabetes drugs already on the market.[27] It is also expensive: about $500 for a three-month supply at the discount Internet price shown in table 5-9. Nonetheless, with aggressive marketing to physicians and plenty of free-sample starter kits, many patients are paying for this more expensive and less effective treatment for initial therapy.

Nonsulfonurea insulin secretagogues (what a mouthful!), such as Starlix and Prandin, are other high-priced diabetes drugs that are similar to the sulfonureas. The two classes are so similar in their method of action, in fact, that they are not recommended to be used together. So if your doctor must choose a drug from one of the two classes, why pick Starlix, at over *twenty-five times* the cost of glipizide? If there is not a good answer, you might request a prescription change. If you are treated for diabetes with any expensive medication and have never tried one of the biguanides or sulfonurea-type drugs, ask your doctor if a substitution would be appropriate, and start saving money.

High Prices for High Blood Pressure

What about drug treatment of hypertension? How do costs vary by class? A newer class, the *angiotensin II receptor blockers* (ARBs), already contains six individual drugs, each introduced by a different pharmaceutical company and each still under patent. Average retail price for ninety days' therapy, at the lowest usual starting dose, ranges from $206 for Cozaar to

$284 for Teveten. So, if an ARB is the best management choice for treatment of your high blood pressure, Cozaar would be the most economical choice.

But compare that to another class of drugs used to treat high blood pressure, the diuretic class. You can buy ninety days' treatment with the diuretic hydrochlorothiazide for less than ten bucks! More important, in almost all clinical trials, diuretics have been unsurpassed in preventing hypertensive heart disease—one of the main reasons you treat high blood pressure in the first place. Diuretics enhance the effects of other drugs if more than one are required for blood pressure control, and they are among the cheapest medicines available. No wonder the NIH's Joint National Committee on Treatment of High Blood Pressure states in its seventh report, "Thiazide-type diuretics should be used as initial therapy for most patients with hypertension . . ." and "diuretics remain underutilized."[27] So why aren't doctors recommending diuretics as a first choice for treatment of hypertension more often? Could it be the pharmaceutical industry's influence on physician prescribing habits?

If you are presently prescribed an overpriced blood pressure pill and nothing else within its class would be a suitable substitute, there are ten or so other classes that may offer a more economical alternative. Respect your doctor's guidance, since some classes may not be appropriate for you. For example, we do not usually recommend beta-blockers for people with asthma or chronic bronchitis, and the use of alpha-1 blockers in older women can worsen urinary incontinence. There are many considerations that go into selection of medications for an individual patient, and you will need your doctor's expertise in determining a suitable regimen for you. Still, make it clear to the physician that cost must be one of those considerations.

TABLE 5-10: Drugs for the Prevention of Migraine Headaches		
Drug class	**Example**	**Price***
Antiepileptic drugs	Topamax (topiramate) 50 mg**	$753
	Depakote ER (divalproex) 500 mg	$241
Calcium-channel blockers	Verapamil, extended release (e.g., Calan SR, Isoptin SR, Covera-HS) 240 mg	$87
Beta-blockers	timolol (Blocadren) 10 mg**	$60
	atenolol (Tenormin) 25 mg	$12
	propranolol (Inderal) 80 mg**	$28
Tricyclic antidepressants	nortriptyline (Pamelor) 25 mg	$19
	desipramine (Norpramin) 25 mg	$31
	amitriptyline (Elavil) 25 mg	$11

* Discount Internet price for a ninety-day supply at the lowest usual recommended starting dose.
** Dosed twice a day.

The Money in Migraines

Several different classes of drugs have been used to prevent frequent, severe, or disabling migraine headaches. (See table 5-10.)* Of the *antiepileptic* drugs used for this purpose, Topamax costs $753 for ninety days' treatment, while Depakote ER costs $241. That's quite a difference. But compare that with another class of drugs to prevent migraines, the tricyclic antidepressants. Of these, a ninety-day supply of nortriptyline costs $19. The beta-blocker class can also prevent migraines

* I am talking about *preventive* therapy here; different classes are used for *intervention* of acute migraine headaches.

for as little as $12 for three months' therapy. Obviously not every migraine sufferer is going to respond to nortriptyline or a beta-blocker, and it is fortunate that we have several drug classes to choose from in order to benefit the greatest number of patients possible. But for initial therapy, why not try the cheapest class first, and leave Topamax—at over sixty times the cost—for the most resistant cases?

Expensive-Drug Survival Index

The most popular expensive drugs are listed alphabetically in the Expensive-Drug Survival Index of this book. Cheaper medicines from alternative classes are listed in the "Alternate-class substitutions" column to the right. Ask your doctor if one of these or a related drug could be substituted as a cost-saving measure. If possible, check prices and be ready to show your doctor how much you would save with the change.

> Say you are taking Requip for restless legs syndrome, but the $261 average retail cost is making your skin crawl and keeping you up at night. Checking the Expensive-Drug Survival Index, we see seven alternative medicines from three different classes that are all standard therapies for RLS. The price for three months' worth of these drugs ranges from around $20 for propoxyphene to $50 for gabapentin. Bringing these price comparisons to your doctor, you could talk about a possible substitution. That $900 in yearly savings makes for a much more restful night's sleep!

You won't always find a cheaper class of medicines for the same treatment goal. If not, the alternate-class substitution column in the survival index will be blank. But if your drug is listed in the index at all, then one of cost-saving methods 10 through 13 will apply. If your drug is not in the index, then perhaps one of the other CSMs will help. Regardless, it never hurts to ask your doctor, "Is there a cheaper class of medicine for the same treatment goal?"

Considerations

Drug therapy can be complex. Often several medications from different classes are required to treat a single condition. Many patients with hypertension will require two or more drugs for blood pressure control. The modern management of congestive heart failure often involves four or five drugs from separate classes. Some medical conditions require drug-class selection that must by highly individualized to the patient. Management of heart arrhythmias and seizure disorders are two such cases; likewise, treatment of AIDS or cancer does not usually permit shopping for the cheapest drug category. In these cases you should rely on your doctor's expertise to determine the most appropriate treatment. Even so, economy can weigh into selection of medication classes; just make sure your doctor knows it's a priority.

Case Study
CSM 12: Use a Cheaper Class of Medicine for the Same Goal

Rochelle is a fifty-six-year-old female nursing-home activities director who transferred into my practice, taking the calcium channel blocker Norvasc for treatment of high blood pressure. This was the first and only drug treatment she had ever been prescribed by her prior physician. The medication was costing her more than $220 every three months, and her blood pressure was still not completely controlled.

Rochelle's blood pressure was brought down to goal with the addition of atenolol, 25 mg daily, but she confided that because she had no health insurance and no prescription benefit, the Norvasc was difficult to afford. We agreed to stop the expensive drug and substitute hydrochlorothiazide, a diuretic costing just pennies per pill.

BEFORE:

Medication	Dose	Cost*
Norvasc	10 mg, 1 daily	$210
Atenolol	25 mg, 1 daily	$12
TOTAL		**$222**

AFTER:

Medication	Dose	Cost*
Hydrochlorothiazide	25 mg, 1/2 daily	$6.50
Atenolol	25 mg, 1 daily	$12
TOTAL		**$18.50**

* Discount Internet price for ninety days' therapy at the patient's prescribed dose.

Rochelle's blood pressure remained under control with the substitution, and her pharmacy costs were reduced to under $75 *per year*. She also got the benefit of using a drug from the diuretic class, medicines that are unsurpassed in preventing heart disease in patients with high blood pressure.

Yearly Savings: $814

Take It to the Bank

- There may be more than one class of medicines available that will treat a medical condition, and some classes are cheaper than others.
- Check the Expensive-Drug Survival Index for each of your costly medicines and note any alternate-class substitutions.
- Compare the price of these drugs with the cost of your present treatment at your pharmacy or an online drugstore.
- Ask your doctor if a substitution is appropriate, and show her the potential savings.
- To keep treatment affordable, always insist that your doctor start with inexpensive drugs from the most economical class.

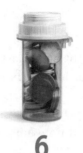

6

Play It Smart!

Cost-Saving Methods 13 through 17

CHAPTER 6 HAS COST-SAVING METHODS that disclose the clever tricks that can save you big bucks. Knowing how to use an online buying service, when to request *fewer* pills from your doctor, and why drug benefit cards make some purchases cost *more* are just some of the tips revealed. You'll also learn to avoid getting new prescriptions for unrecognized side effects and why your doctor *needs* to give away drugs for free. Read on to discover these and more money-saving tips, and start playing it smart!

CSM 13: Cut Costs by Splitting Tablets

Cutting tablets in half can also cut drug costs in half. If you are prescribed a single 20 mg tablet of Lipitor daily, taking half of a 40 mg tablet will cost you half as much. This is because the 20 and 40 mg strengths are priced the same; so is the 80 mg strength. Apparently, Lipitor's manufacturer wants all patients taking Lipitor to incur the same cost whether they take the 20, 40, or 80 mg tablet. This is called *flat pricing.*

Many other drugs cost the same regardless of tablet strength. When higher strength pills do cost more (called *graduated pricing*), the higher strengths are usually discounted so that the cost per milligram is still less. The US Department of Veterans Affairs knows this. In one study, a group from the VA saved over half a million dollars by splitting tablets.[1] Unfortunately, most MDs are oblivious to drug pricing, so don't expect your doctor to prescribe half tablets. Remember, when it comes to prescribing economy, you will need to educate your doctor.

Is there a downside to splitting tablets? Well, the uniformity of tablets can be a concern. If the active ingredient is not distributed evenly throughout the tablet, the amount of medicine in each of two halves could be different, even if you manage to split them perfectly. Splitting tablets evenly can be difficult too, depending on your vision, coordination, or mental state, and depending on the shape and form of the pill. Studies show that even pharmacy technicians can't always cut them straight down the middle.[2]

Proof in the Pudding

But the proof of the pudding is always in the eating. If the treatment still works, then it doesn't matter if the active ingredient is unevenly distributed or if the cut isn't perfect. Two studies of more than two thousand patients who changed to split tablets for six or more weeks showed no detrimental changes in treatment for cholesterol.[3] Another study of patients taking either whole or split doses of lisinopril showed no significant differences in lowering of their blood pressure.[4]

Many tablets are scored, notched, or indented by the manufacturer for ease of splitting. The FDA approves these formulations after some additional testing. Pill-splitting devices—available in most drugstores for under $10—can help. Of course, bigger, elongated, and deeply scored tablets are easiest to split. Small, smooth, spherical, or odd-shaped tablets are more difficult to sever evenly. Capsules and "gelcaps" should not be split at all. Enteric-coated* and extended-release tablets should not usually be split, although there are exceptions (for example, Toprol-XL is scored for splitting). Also, certain combination tablets containing two drugs, such as Vytorin (ezetemibe/simvistatin), should not be split since the dose of one of the two medicines (in this case ezetemibe) is not recommended at half strength. Therefore, you should check with your doctor or pharmacist about the suitability of splitting any particular medication tablet.

---

* *Enteric-coated* is a term that refers to an outer layer or covering on a tablet that delays dissolution until it passes through the stomach and into the intestine.

Split Decision

Now that you know about the potential savings, how are you going to find out if tablet splitting will work for you? You could just ask your doctor at your treatment review visit, or you could scout ahead. You will always help your cause more by proposing a specific change and showing the savings. Many popular drugs are listed in the Expensive-Drug Survival Index of this book. Medications suitable for splitting are indicated by an "S" in the second column to the right. (Of course, if you are taking the highest available strength of any tablet, splitting will not apply.) If your expensive drug is not listed, available tablet strengths can be found in the *Physician's Desk Reference* (PDR) and other pharmacy reference books or on most online drugstore websites. Look for a strength twice the dose of yours in tablet form. Find for the best price and bring the savings information to your doctor.

As long as the desired treatment is not compromised, splitting tablets is a convenient way to save big on pharmacy costs. Slight variations in split tablet size usually don't matter. I reassure nervous pill-splitters by telling them to take the "big half" now and the "small half" next dose. That way, any variations in dose are compensated for with the next half tablet. We then follow the treatment to make sure that blood pressure, cholesterol, depression, or whatever their condition may be, remains well treated. If the precise medication dose is not critical to the therapeutic effect, and if the drug has a long duration of action (as most once- or twice-a-day medicines do), any differences in portion sizes of split tablets is usually inconsequential. Table 6-1 shows the cost savings from splitting some of the more commonly prescribed drugs.

TABLE 6-1: Whole- and Split-Tablet Prices of Ten Popular Drugs			
Medication	**Whole-tablet price***	**Price of equivalent dose split tablet***	**Three-month savings (%)**
Lipitor	$425 (20 mg)	$212.50 (1/2 x 40 mg)	$212.50 (50%)
Toprol XL	$99 (25 mg)	$49.50 (1/2 x 50 mg)	$49.50 (50%)
Norvasc	$208 (5 mg)	$139.50 (1/2 x 10 mg)	$63.50 (31%)
Lexapro	$298 (10 mg)	$155.50 (1/2 x 20 mg)	$142.50 (48%)
Diovan	$221 (80 mg)	$119.00 (1/2 x 160 mg)	$102.00 (46%)
Crestor	$354 (10 mg)	$177.00 (1/2 x 20 mg)	$177.00 (50%)
Actos	$403 (15 mg)	$222.50 (1/2 x 30 mg)	$80.50 (20%)
Altace	$197 (5 mg)	$115.50 (1/2 x 10 mg)	$81.50 (44%)
Cozaar	$206 (50 mg)	$140.50 (1/2 x 100 mg)	$65.50 (32%)
Viagra	$448 (50 mg, #30)	$224.00 (1/2 x 100 mg, #15)	$224.00 (50%)

* Average retail price for a ninety-day supply.

Take It to the Bank

- Check the strength of each of your medications against other available strengths (either with your doctor, in a pharmacy reference such as the *Physician's Desk Reference* [PDR], or on a drugstore website such as Familymeds. com.) Is a double-strength tablet available that can be split?
- Some of your medicines may be listed in the Expensive-Drug Survival Index of this book. If so, those that come

in tablets suitable for splitting are indicated by an "S" in the second column.

- Ask your doctor to prescribe double-strength tablets at half-tablet dosing whenever appropriate.
- Always use a pill-splitting device to improve uniformity.
- Follow-up with your doctor to ensure consistent response to treatment.

CSM 14: Get It Prescribed Right!

A little bit of knowledge of medication dosing and pricing can allow you to continue the identical medication at the exact same dosage at savings of 75 percent or more. How? Get it prescribed to your best advantage.

How Many Do I Take?

Few patients or physicians are aware that different available strengths of a particular medication are often sold at or near the same price, a practice called flat pricing. As we learned with cost-saving method 13, the 20 mg, 40 mg, and 80 mg strengths of the cholesterol-lowering drug Lipitor all retail at nearly the same price. Thus, a ninety-day supply of Lipitor taken as a single 80 mg tablet per day—instead of two 40 mg tablets—would cut the cost from $850 to $425. I pity the unfortunate patient prescribed four 20 mg Lipitor tablets per day. It's still 80 mg, but at a cost of over $6,800 a year. Ouch!

Recently, I met someone taking multiple capsules of the medication Neurontin, prescribed in a way that needlessly increased her cost. She was taking four 100 mg capsules twice a day at a cost of $572 every three months. What she didn't know was that a single 400 mg capsule taken twice daily costs $428 over the same period, a savings of $576 per year.

It isn't surprising that patients arrive at such impractical doses. Neurontin is a medicine that is typically increased gradually over a few weeks' time to minimize side effects and determine the lowest effective dose. This patient's neurologist had started her on 100 mg a day and gradually increased the dose week by week. She was given a large supply of 100 mg capsules to start but continued to take the lower-strength capsules even after arriving at her optimal dose.

This is the typical scenario for drugs dosed two or more at a time. The treatment starts with one pill but is increased at subsequent office visits until an effective dose is reached. Since the patient already has the medicine, she is instructed to take two (or more) of the medicine on hand rather than buy a new prescription of higher strength pills. This makes sense at the time, because it is still uncertain what dose will be required. But few patients realize that, once the best dose is determined, there may be a cheaper way to get it than taking multiple pills.

If you are taking more than one at a time of any tablet or capsule, find out what other strengths of that medicine are available. There may be a higher-strength pill that would equal your present dose, at a significantly lower price. Are you taking two 75 mg Effexor XR a day? Buying the 150 mg tablets would save you over $1,500 a year. Has your doctor increased your 25 mg Toprol-XL dose to two tablets daily? You might want to know that the 25 mg and 50 mg tablets both retail for about a dollar per pill. So the 50 mg strength saves you 50 percent on every prescription, or $365 per year.

You can find out all of the available strengths for each medicine you take in a drug reference book, from your pharmacy, or at any number of websites. Finding your medicine on an online drugstore's website (CVS.com, Familymeds.com) is especially informative because all the available strengths are listed, along with the relative retail prices. If you discover a more economical way to get the same medication and dose, write down the information and potential savings for discussion with your doctor.

How Often Do I Take It?

Learning the usual dosing interval or frequency of each of your medications can also lead to better prescribing efficiency and economy. Consider the patient who was prescribed the blood pressure medication Norvasc by his cardiologist at a dose of 5 mg daily. It helped, but when blood pressure readings were not quite to goal, the doctor increased the dose to 5 mg twice a day. This controlled his blood pressure, but he complained to me about the $400 cost for a three-month prescription. Knowing that Norvasc has a long duration of action and is usually dosed once daily (no matter the strength of the tablet), I suggested that he get the 10 mg tablets and take one a day. With his cardiologist's approval, he made the change and happily reported more than $125 in savings on every prescription refill.

Going Broke Drop by Drop

I don't need to tell anyone taking prescription eye drops that these medications can be as expensive as any others. A 2.5 ml bottle of the most widely prescribed glaucoma medicine, Xalatan, contains 50 to 70 drops and retails for $78 on average; that's over a dollar per drop! If your ophthalmologist prescribes two drops at a time, your savings can trickle away fast. But a little knowledge about the eye can plug unnecessary leaks in your bank account. According to the *Medical Letter on Drugs and Therapeutics*, the average volume of a drop of eye medicine is 35 to 50 microliters. Well, a human eye even brimming with fluid only holds 30 microliters, so even one drop is an overdose. A second drop either overflows to the face or down the tear duct and into the nose. That expensive solution in your nose probably does little good for your eye, but it *doubles* the cost of therapy and increases the chance of side effects. Eye specialist consultants to the *Medical Letter* agreed that ". . . all eye drops should generally be given as one drop," a practice that will save patients 50 percent on their eye prescriptions.[5]

Playing the Insurance Game

Silly insurance rules can also needlessly cost you money. Consider Emile, who was prescribed hydrochlorothiazide (HCT) for high blood pressure at a dose of a half tablet every morning. Insurance rules allowed only one month of medicine to be filled at a time. So every month Emile would go to the pharmacy to pick up his fifteen tablets, paying the minimum plan co-payment of $10. So the medication was costing him $120 per year. Well, guess what? You can buy a year's supply of HCT for $10! By using his insurance prescription plan, Emile's out-of-pocket expense was *ten times higher* than the retail cost. You would think the pharmacist would have alerted him to this absurdity, but not so. I told Emile that the next time he went to fill a prescription for HCT, he should get a year's supply, and leave his insurance card—*and* an extra $100—in his wallet.

This example again illustrates the pitfalls of going, prescription in hand, to the pharmacy without any knowledge of how much the medicine should cost. Those with prescription plans often feel reassured by fairly reasonable co-payments. "It can't be any worse than $55," they tell themselves. Well, how would you feel about paying $55 for a nonformulary prescription that retails for $1.85? "Cheated" is the word that comes to my mind. Before using any prescription coverage, *always* find out what the drug costs retail. Then you can choose the most economical way of paying for it.

How Many Are You Giving Me?

"I stopped the new prescription, doctor. It was making me sick." Mr. Lawrence had returned to my office two weeks after beginning the new treatment for hypertension. It is not unusual for some patients to be intolerant of a new medicine, and I explained that we would need to try something else to control his blood pressure. "What do I do with the eighty-seven pills I have left over? They cost me $75 and the drugstore won't take 'em back!"

Oops. Mr. Lawrence's irritation was justified. I had written the new prescription for the usual three-month supply of medication in good faith, expecting that it would lower his pressure safely without problems. It had performed well for many of my other patients. Now I could only apologize for the cost of the remaining unusable tablets. That embarrassing incident taught me one of the lessons of this chapter: accepting a prescription for more than a few weeks' worth of a new medicine is a needless risk to your pocketbook.

When your doctor writes a prescription for new long-term treatment, ask for no more than a few weeks' worth of medicine, just enough to give it a reasonable trial. That way, if you experience intolerable side effects, or if the medicine just does not work, you will not have a big bottle of useless pills left over. If the medicine performs adequately, you can then get a prescription for a larger amount.

This principle can also apply to one-time prescriptions. How many of us have paid dearly for a generous supply of medicine for a problem that resolves after one or two doses? Do we really need sixty pain pills for an ankle sprain? Why get thirty or forty tranquilizers for one round-trip airplane flight? We could blame the doctors for overestimating the number of pills needed, but it is time for patients to start looking after their own prescription expenditures.

How many sleeping pills do you think you will use to get though a period of temporary, stress-related insomnia? Once a prescription is agreed upon, tell the doctor how many pills you would like prescribed. If she disagrees with your request, she will let you know. But if you say you want ten, she certainly isn't going to give you thirty, and you will have saved 66 percent on the cost.

How many days' worth of pain pills do you need following an injury? Your doctor will have an idea of the range and may tend to prescribe even beyond that estimate. (He wants to keep extra phone calls for refill requests to a minimum.) Ask for half that number of pills, with an available refill, or a third as many with two refills. Then you can always get more medication if needed without disrupting the doctor, and you won't buy a larger quantity than you will use.

Take It to the Bank

- If you are taking more than one of any pill at a time, find out what other strengths of the drug are available. You may be able to get an equal dose of the same medication in a single higher-dose tablet at a much lower cost. Convey the potential cost savings to your doctor. Whenever medication dosing is doubled, ask whether higher-strength pills could be substituted.
- If you are taking any drug more than once a day, find out its recommended dosing interval. You may be able to get an equal daily amount administered in a single higher-dose tablet at a much lower cost.
- Because the eye can only hold one drop of medication, instilling a second drop doubles your prescription cost with no therapeutic benefit. Using one drop instead of two cuts prescription eye-drop costs in half.
- Always find out the retail price of a prescription before using a prescription drug insurance plan. Only use the

insurance plan if the out-of-pocket cost (the co-payment) is less than the drug's retail price.

- Only accept a few weeks' supply of a newly prescribed medicine for long-term treatment. That way, if the treatment is not satisfactory, you will not have paid for a large supply of unusable pills.

- For temporary treatments taken on an as-needed basis, request fewer pills (with available refills). This will help you avoid buying many more pills than you will use.

CSM 15: Don't Treat Side Effects of One Drug with Another

The first rule of pharmacology is: every drug has more than one effect. There is the effect you want—the one the medicine is prescribed for—and then there are the other actions of the drug, the side effects. These are the hastily recited, sometimes alarming, often comical, possible adverse consequences given at the end of those annoying TV ads for prescription drugs. How the marketers can assume that we will all rush to our doctors requesting medications that are going to result in oily anal discharge is beyond me!

One Bad Drug Deserves Another?

Whether it is recognized or not, thousands of prescriptions are written each year to treat the side effects of another medication. There are cases where this is considered sound, standard medical practice. Prescribing potassium for patients taking diuretics is an example. Treating nausea associated with cancer chemotherapy or general anesthetics is also certainly justified.

The issue is a bit trickier when a patient taking medications presents to his doctor with a common complaint such as cough, muscle aches, depressed mood, sexual dysfunction, or a rash. She may already be on an intricate regimen of several medications that has been fine-tuned with great perseverance. Is the new symptom a side effect of one of the medicines or is it a symptom of a new medical problem? It can take a great deal of patience to sort this out. We don't want to upset the therapy, but neither do we want to order unnecessary tests or prescribe additional medication because of a side effect. For any new, unexplained symptoms occurring in a patient taking medications, adverse reaction to medications must be considered. Otherwise, a new prescription aimed at the symptoms may follow, adding to the expense of therapy and risking even more side effects.

Imagine a woman taking birth control pills who develops high blood pressure. A new prescription is added that controls her blood pressure well but is complicated by development of a depression. Counseling doesn't help, and she is started on an antidepressant. This in turn results in insomnia. Now a sedative is prescribed. Not only is this woman's care medically poor, her pharmacy bills will make her *financially* poor as well! Of course she could stop all of the treatments and try a different contraceptive, which would probably solve all of her symptoms.

Below are examples of common medication side effects that are often mistaken for new medical problems and treated with additional prescriptions.

Cough

Chronic cough is a ubiquitous symptom that may be caused by lung diseases, allergies, or even digestive disorders. It is also a common side effect of *angiotensin converting enzyme* (ACE) inhibitors. ACE inhibitors—which include Accupril (quinapril), Aceon (perindopril), Altace (ramipril), Capoten (captopril), Lotensin (benazepril), Mavik (trandolapril), Monopril (fosinopril), Prinivil/Zestril (lisinopril), Univasc (moexipril), and Vasotec (enalapril)—are a popular and effective treatment for high blood pressure, congestive heart failure, diabetic kidney disease, and other conditions. Up to 30 percent of patients taking ACE inhibitors will develop a nagging cough, throat clearing, a tickle in the throat, or laryngeal swelling. Unfortunately, too many of these patients are misdiagnosed and started on treatment for asthma, stomach acid reflux, or postnasal drip. The asthma inhaler Flovent ($102 per month), the allergy drug Singulair ($126 per month), and the acid blocker Prevacid ($186 per month) can be excellent treatments, unless you don't need them. In that case, they are a substantial drain on resources. Do you have the ACE inhibitor cough? If so, a change of therapy is the best way to remedy this annoying side effect.

Erectile Dysfunction

Almost any blood pressure pill and most medications for depression can cause sexual side effects. But did you know that statin drugs to lower cholesterol increase the incidence of erectile dysfunction in men by 50 percent?[6] Considering Lipitor, Zocor, and Pravachol are the second, twelfth, and forty-second most-often-prescribed drugs in the United States, that's a lot of dysfunction.* Potency drugs Viagra, Levitra, or Cialis could be prescribed, but at \$15 to \$17 a pill, it's an expensive proposition. Why not stop the offending agent instead? If several drugs are being taken and it is uncertain which might be causing a side effect, a sequential holiday from each will usually reveal it. A list of your medications in order of most likely offender to least should be made by your doctor. Then each drug is stopped sequentially for a week or so, in the order given, until you find the culprit. Then go back to your doctor for a change in therapy. Only do this in conjunction with your physician. ***Warning:*** *You must be slowly weaned off some antihypertension medicines to prevent a rebound of very high blood pressure.*

Rashes

Sequential drug holidays may need to be outlined for those developing a rash. It makes little sense—and should be considered poor practice—to only treat an allergic drug rash with salves, antihistamines, or steroids when stopping the offending drug will cure the problem. Needless to say, it is also much cheaper.

---

* Other side effects of statin drugs include peripheral neuropathy, memory loss, sleep disturbances, lupus-like syndrome, male breast development, and pancreatitis.[7]

Mood Disturbances

It is my practice to take newly, mildly depressed patients off of beta-blocking drugs or oral contraceptives before considering them for antidepressant therapy with medication, especially if the mood disturbance appears after these drugs are started. A change of therapy is often all that is needed to correct the depression and saves the patient the expense of antidepressant medicines. It also avoids more side effects from the antidepressants.

Heartburn

Heartburn is a common malady in our society. Strolling down that long drugstore aisle stacked high with antacids betrays our digestive weakness. Rolaids, Tums, Maalox, Mylanta, Zantac, Pepcid, Tagamet, and Zegerid wait, ready to relieve common indigestion. No wonder it is easy to overlook the osteoporosis drugs Fosamax, Actonel, and Boniva as a cause of one's heartburn. The makers of these agents have conducted an intensive campaign to let patients and physicians know of the risk of inflammation, erosions, ulcerations, or strictures of the esophagus with their products. They have incorporated specific instructions on the manner of administration in order to minimize these adverse reactions. Still, women taking these drugs are too often prescribed acid-blocking drugs like Nexium and Protonix to combat the side effects, when the proper course is to stop the offending agent.

Muscle Aches

What doctor's office complaint could be more typical than muscle aches? Muscular aches and pains are a part of life. They are also a common side effect of many cholesterol-lowering drugs. With the stricter guidelines for cholesterol management and increasing use of statin drugs, new complaints of muscle aches had better be investigated carefully. The statins include Crestor, Lescol, Lipitor, lovastatin, Pravachol, and Zocor (simvistatin). All are known to cause muscle pain and inflammation (myopathy). Although this occurs in only one in twenty patients taking these drugs, continuing the medicine can result in muscle cell destruction leading to kidney failure. So not only can treatment of statin-induced myopathy with anti-inflammatory drugs, muscle relaxants, or pain relievers be expensive, it can also be dangerous. Taking statins in combination with many other popular drugs (including warfarin, digoxin, certain antibiotics, and the fibrates gemfibrozil and Tricor) makes the risk of myopathy even more common.[8] Even so, the cause of the resulting symptoms may go unrecognized. Patients taking statins should be warned and questioned regarding new or unexplained muscle aches, and the medication withdrawn when appropriate.

Case Study
CSM 15: Don't Treat Side Effects of One Drug with Another

Fumiko is a retired housekeeper with high blood pressure who came in complaining of depression that had been worsening for several months. She had battled depression years before and had responded to a course of therapy with Lexapro. Treatment of her blood pressure included the beta-blocker metoprolol, a medication that can cause or worsen depression.[9] Although it was tempting to restart treatment with Lexapro, we instead agreed to change metoprolol to another agent. By the time Fumiko returned to the office two weeks later, her depression had completely resolved! The new medicine kept her blood pressure controlled without side effects. By considering her medications as a possible cause of new symptoms, treatment of a side effect of one drug with another drug was avoided.

Yearly Savings: $1,192

Take It to the Bank

- Recall or ask your doctor the indication for each medication you take. Could any have been started in treatment of a side effect of another medication?
- Always be suspicious of new symptoms that begin after you start a new medication, especially cough, sexual disorders, rashes, muscle aches, depression, or heartburn.
- Ask if drugs causing and treating side effects can be stopped, with appropriate follow-up as necessary.

CSM 16: Shop!

Say you have a newly written prescription from your doctor that you plan to fill at one of the local drugstores. What do you think the variation in cost might be among nearby retailers? Fifteen percent? Twenty percent at the most? If you're thinking that the few dollars saved at the pharmacy across town won't even cover the cost of the extra gas consumed to get there, how wrong you might be. That prescription may cost over *three times* more at one drugstore compared to the next! But if you don't shop, you'll never know how much you could save.

Let Your Fingers Do It

A while back, I prescribed a one-month supply of fluoxetine 40 mg capsules (generic Prozac) to a patient without prescription drug coverage. I was surprised when she called the next day requesting a cheaper medicine. It seems that our local Longs Drugs wanted more than $150 for the prescription. "Over $5 a pill for generic fluoxetine!" I blurted into the phone in disbelief. "That can't be right." So I called up Longs and asked them myself. Sure enough, their price for thirty of the 40 mg capsules was $152.95. (The same amount of Prozac, the brand-name version, was priced at $334!) Then I called Sav-On. They wanted $119 for the same prescription—a little better. So I called my patient back and told her that before changing medicines she should call around to see who had the best price for fluoxetine, since there did seem to be some variation. The results of her shopping—which consisted of making five local telephone calls—astounded me. They are summarized in table 6-2.

TABLE 6-2: Quoted Price for Thirty Generic 40 mg Fluoxetine Capsules at Various North San Luis Obispo County Drugstores, April 2006					
Drugstore	Longs Drugs	Rite Aid	Sav-On Drugs	Walgreens	Wal-Mart
Quoted price	$152.95	$124.99	$119.00	$79.99	$41.36

The price difference for a month's supply of generic Prozac at local drugstores varied by over $110! These retailers are all within a few miles of each other. How could some drugstores possibly justify the markup in price? I do not mean for table 6-2 to indicate that drug prices are always lower at Walgreen's than at Longs Drugs, or that Sav-On is always more expensive than Wal-Mart. Prices vary among the retailers from drug to drug. A patient recently informed me that her blood pressure prescription is cheaper at Rite Aid than at Walgreen's, quite the opposite from their pricing of fluoxetine. So you have to shop for the best deal on each medication you take, even if it means using different pharmacies for different drugs.

My mother, who never forgot her Great Depression–era upbringing, buys certain grocery staples at one supermarket, but her meats at a different store. She may even pick up produce at yet another market. She likes all of the stores, but some have better deals on some goods than the others. It's called shopping. Americans are usually very talented when it comes to finding the best deal for most expenditures, especially big-ticket items. But for some reason, this does not always carry over to drug prescriptions. Why don't people shop when it comes to prescription drugs? The price for an equivalent prescription—the same amount of the same drug by the same manufacturer—can vary widely from pharmacy to pharmacy. You will always save more by buying each expensive drug at the specific pharmacy offering the best deal. Hopefully, after applying the cost-saving methods, you will be left with no more than one or two costlier drugs and can limit purchases to as many pharmacies. But you still must call around for the best price.

Quantity Matters

The price of certain prescription medicines also can vary with the number of pills purchased. A patient of mine without prescription benefits was calling around (shopping) for the best price on her medicines. She reported to me that the local Wal-Mart sold thirty atenolol 25 mg tablets for $11.62, about 39 cents per tablet. But they also sold sixty of the very same tablets for just $13.68, about 23 cents per tablet! That's a 40 percent discount just for buying thirty more tablets. Granted, atenolol is not an expensive drug and the savings here are meager, but this illustrates that you can get a price break on medications depending on the quantity purchased. Just find out what number of pills gives you the best deal. If you discover that 90, 100, 360—or whatever the quantity—sells at a substantially cheaper price per pill, tell your doctor that is the number you would like, and start enjoying those savings.

As my patient and I discovered, shopping among local drugstores can save 70 percent or more, and buying in quantity can save an additional 40 percent. If you then expand your shopping sphere to include nationwide mail-order and online retailers, you can save even more.

Let Your Mouse Do It

Driving to a local drugstore can be convenient, especially if you need to pick up some toothpaste, cat food, or the latest issue of *Hot Rod* magazine along with your prescription. But when you consider the exorbitant prices of some medications these days, doing so can be financially careless. If you are taking medication on a regular basis and have not investigated online mail-order pharmacies, it's time to get started. Just because you don't routinely drive past these retailers doesn't mean they are not a trustworthy and reliable source for your medication purchases. Prices tend to be much lower than retail drugstores can offer, and the competition among them works further to your advantage. Table 6-3 shows comparison prices for five popular medicines at five US-based online mail-order pharmacies. Compare them with the average retail price listed and what you may be paying at a local drugstore.

TABLE 6-3: Average Retail and Online Mail-Order Prices (Including Shipping) for Five Common Drugs*					
	Lipitor 20 mg tabs	**lisinopril 10 mg tabs**	**Protonix 40 mg caps**	**metform-in 500 mg tabs****	**Lexapro 10 mg tabs**
Average retail price	$425	$93	$426	$131	$298
Costco.com*** 1-800-774-2678	$342	$10	$342	$20	$229
Drugstore.com 1-800-378-4786	$336	$32	$352	$56	$229
RxUSA.com 1-800-764-3648	$350	$34	$375	$42	$233
CVS.com 1-888-607-4287	$382	$38	$367	$55	$244
FamilyMeds.com 1-888-787-2800	$320	$31	$350	$56	$226

   * For a ninety-day supply at usual dosing.
  ** Dosed twice a day.
 *** Calculated from advertised 100-pill rate.

Although online pharmacy prices are generally much better than the average retail price, there is still some variation among them. Ninety 20 mg Lipitor tablets sell for $382 at CVS.com, while the same amount from FamilyMeds.com is $320—a 16 percent savings. So even shopping among the mail-order pharmacies can pay off. If you don't want to visit the websites of each of the online retailers above to compare prices, an online shopping service can do it for you! DestinationRx.com is just such a service that provides prices of prescription drugs from each of the vendors listed in table 6-3. Simply enter the name of the drug you take, click on a quantity, and the relative prices at several of the vendors are revealed. There are direct links to the pharmacy websites, so you can order your medication at the best price right then and there.

The pharmacy websites will take you through the process of ordering, creating an account, and verifying your prescription. You can mail a doctor's written prescription to them, have your doctor call or fax them, or they will call your doctor—just like at your neighborhood drugstore. You can pay with a credit card and can use insurance or discount cards. Like any pharmacy, they will create and keep a health profile of your medical problems, medications, allergies, and so on. Shipping is usually free for larger orders and requires some time, so you must reorder before your supplies are completely depleted.

Security

Any pharmacy you buy from should be accredited, including online retailers. In response to public concern about the safety of pharmacy practices on the Internet, the National Association of Boards of Pharmacy (NABP) developed the Verified Internet Pharmacy Practice Sites (VIPPS) program in the spring of 1999. To be VIPPS accredited, a pharmacy must comply with the licensing and inspection requirements of its state and each state to which it dispenses pharmaceuticals. In addition, accredited pharmacies must demonstrate compliance with VIPPS criteria to the NABP, including patient rights to privacy, authentication and security of prescription orders, adherence to a recognized quality-assurance policy, and provision of meaningful consultation between patients and pharmacists. A VIPPS-accredited pharmacy is identified by the VIPPS hyperlink seal displayed on its website. By clicking on the seal, you are linked to the NABP VIPPS site (http://vipps.nabp.net/verify.asp). Here, you can verify an online pharmacy as accredited simply by entering its web address (URL) in the space provided and clicking the "verify" button. *It is my recommendation that you only purchase medications online from verified Internet pharmacy sites.*

But I Don't Have Internet Access!

If you don't have Internet access readily available, the toll-free telephone numbers are also provided for each of the online vendors in table 6-3. These are all VIPPS accredited retailers. Give them a call and inquire about pricing just as you would with any local drugstore.

Cross the Border

Presently, it is illegal to reimport prescription drugs, yet $1.5 billion of them are shipped into the United States for personal use from foreign vendors each year, half of that from Canada. That's a lot of unimpeded criminal activity. Apparently border officials and the US Post Office are overlooking most of these felonies. Patients have told me that some of their Canadian pharmacy shipments have been confiscated at the border, but most shipments continue unchecked. I am not about to suggest that you break the law to get your drugs cheaper. But if enough people think a law is wrong, then perhaps it is not justified. Maybe some drug reimportation laws could be repealed. I understand that a number of states and localities have encouraged government employees to buy imported drugs in defiance of federal law. *

Domestic or foreign, you should only purchase prescription drugs from accredited vendors. Unfortunately, VIPPS has refused to certify Canadian pharmacies that sell to US customers, and the FDA is not willing to work with the Canadian International Pharmacy Association (CIPA) to certify legitimate online pharmacies. So if you want to verify accreditation of a foreign online pharmacy, it will need to come from independent agencies unaffiliated with the US government. Below are descriptions of a few entities verifying Canadian and other foreign online retailers. Each has a characteristic seal that appears on the home pages of participating websites. The more such seals you see on a particular site, the more

* Illinois, Kansas, Missouri, Wisconsin, and Vermont formed a cartel to buy prescription drugs from pharmacies in Ireland, Britain, and Canada. That program, at Isaverx.net, requires some sixty approved pharmacies abroad to meet each state's own safety rules and regulations for dispensing prescription drugs.

surveillance, verification, and accreditation of the online retailer there is, and the more assurance you have of a safe purchase. Just like at home, all such pharmacies require a prescription from your physician. *It is foolhardy to buy medications from foreign vendors that do not require a prescription, do not have a licensed pharmacist on site, do not have a verifiable land-based address, and do not offer any kind of certification, accreditation, or licensure from an authoritative body.*

PC

PharmacyChecker.com LLC (PC) is the leading independent source of information about online pharmacies. PC collects, evaluates, and reports on credentials, prices, and customer feedback. It helps consumers find the lowest-priced products from the most qualified and reputable online pharmacies. It also provides market intelligence and publishes pharmacy ratings, profiles, and drug-price comparisons online at www.pharmacychecker.com.

CIPA

The Canadian International Pharmacy Association (CIPA) represents legitimate and licensed Canadian pharmacies that provide international services. CIPA was created in 2002 to promote the growth and viability of Canadian pharmacies, and to ensure the highest standards of practice by its members. Pharmacies' membership can be verified on the CIPA website at www.ciparx.ca.

NAPAC

The North American Pharmacy Accreditation Commission (NAPAC) was founded to assist consumers in selecting reputable online pharmacies in all of North America. Membership of participating pharmacies and specific health care sites is based upon recognized Standards of Practices Guidelines enforced by the NAPAC Executive Committee. These standards include customer service, quality of product, receipt of goods via US mail and/or Canada post, confirmed (verifiable) pharmacist licensure in the United States and/or Canada, and expedited resolution of complaints. NAPAC operates as an independent organization and is not funded by pharmaceutical manufacturers, major retail pharmacy chains, and/or government agencies. NAPAC answers to no one but the consumer. The NAPAC Seal is retained by participating member sites.

IMPAC

The Internet and Mail-Order Pharmacy Accreditation Commission (IMPAC) defines quality and safety standards for mail-order and Internet pharmacies. The commission verifies adherence to standards and provides certification for international pharmacies in the United States, Canada, and other countries. Accredited pharmacies display the IMPAC seal on their websites.

Take It to the Bank

- Prices for medications among local drugstores can vary considerably, even 300 to 400 percent. So it pays to shop.

- There is often a price break on medications depending on the quantity purchased. Always ask what quantity provides the best value, and ask your doctor to prescribe that amount.
- Nationwide mail-order and online retailers offer even better prices and make sense for those taking medications on an ongoing basis.
- Although widely done, it is presently illegal to have medications shipped to you from foreign pharmacies.
- You should only purchase prescription drugs from accredited vendors, regardless of whether they are domestic or foreign.
- It is foolhardy to buy medications from foreign vendors that do not require a prescription, do not have a licensed pharmacist on site, do not have a verifiable land-based address, and do not offer any kind of certification, accreditation, or licensure from an authoritative body.

CSM 17: Get It for Free

In chapter 5 I warned against beginning *new* long-term treatment with drug-company samples. However, a free handout of an expensive drug you *must* take is just like money in your pocket—for a while.

Let me say right off, you cannot win at this game. Eventually, at some point, you will end up paying for the stuff. Your doctor might give you samples to last several months, maybe a year or more, but one fateful day the drug company piper will need to be paid. Therefore, this method should be a temporary one used to hold you over until some other means of obtaining the essential drug is found. Other possibilities are the subject of cost-saving methods 18 through 20.

My father-in-law, Chester, was always bragging about never having to pay for his medicine. His doctor had generously loaded him up with sacks of free-sample bottles of Lotrel when he was first diagnosed with high blood pressure. It seemed that at every office visit he was given more free samples. A year passed before he finally got to the last of the little plastic vials containing a few fancy tablets in each. Overall, he received more than $1,000 of free medicine, but at long last, the doctor's supplies ran out. I'll never forget his dismay the day he came back from the drugstore after having to actually buy Lotrel for the first time. "Three hundred dollars," he grumbled, "for ninety pills!" Game over—you lose. Suddenly, the free sample deal wasn't so praiseworthy. I told him (in my loving way) to quit complaining and either foot the bill for the treatment or ask his doctor to prescribe something cheaper.

This scenario is not rare. Perhaps you recognize yourself in the same situation: the sample pills are great while they last, but when the well runs dry, you quickly find that the cost for a prescription is outrageous. But this outcome is predictable. The drug companies aren't going to keep giving away free medicine. The samples are provided to conveniently get you started on a long-term, costly, and patented product that you will need to buy later. Nobody is giving your doctor inexpensive generic medicines to dole out. Just the fact that your doctor has free samples should be a warning: "DANGER: EXPENSIVE MEDICATION."

In a special communication to the *Journal of the American Medical Association* (*JAMA*) in January 2006, eleven doctors with affiliations with the most prestigious academic medical centers across the country stated, "The availability of free samples is a powerful inducement for physicians and patients to rely on medications that are expensive but not more effective."[10]

You may have noticed that many of the cost-saving methods steer you away from the type of drugs that are sampled to your doctor. These aggressively marketed products are usually going to be a poor value. Most are the overpriced, redundant drugs described earlier. You would be better served if none of your prescription medications are even in your doctor's free-giveaway drug cabinet. Trick-or-treating for drugs is the least reliable cost-saving method and a strategy to be used only under the following circumstances:

1. Your condition absolutely requires treatment with a drug that is sampled to your doctor's office, *and*
2. You are in the process of getting assistance through a government, pharmacy benefit, or drug-company program (CSMs 18 through 20), *or*
3. You are undergoing treatment for a condition with a finite course of therapy, such as antibiotics for an infection or acid blockers for an ulcer.

So, unless it is a temporary situation, you should always investigate what less-expensive, alternative treatment could be tried before you resort to the sample-giveaway scam. If there is something cheaper that can also do the job, you will save money in the long run, even if samples seem plentiful for now.

Still, though temporary, substantial savings can be realized with free drug samples. Sometimes the best treatment for your situation may just happen to be an expensive brand-name product. Perhaps you are taking a genuine breakthrough drug that is still under patent. What can you do if it is not affordable?

Stock Up!

Here is how the drug companies' marketing scheme can work to your advantage: Drug manufacturers want your doctor to think of using their product first. One method they use is to send sales representatives (*drug reps*) to every doctor's office in America with trunkloads of their newest (and costliest) drugs. Free drug samples worth more than $10 billion were provided to doctors' offices in 2001 alone.[11] These inextricably packaged pills (sometimes one per box) are designed to attract the eye of a physician rummaging through the sample cupboard. And the more boxes provided—and shelf space occupied—the better they serve their purpose: to sublimely habituate the doctor into starting as many patients as possible on their drug. Sampled medications are usually the ones prescribed for long-term therapy, such as for treatment of high blood pressure, high cholesterol, or diabetes—medications that may be continued for years. So it's a big deal to the company which drug your doctor chooses. If it's that company's product, its ongoing sales and profits are assured until the patent expires (or the patient's money runs out).

A physician who considers, for example, all angiotensin receptor blockers (ARBs) to be roughly equivalent in treating high blood pressure is very likely to start a patient on new therapy with whatever samples are available in his cabinet. Say there are many Diovan samples sitting there, taking up a whole shelf, but just a handful of Cozaar. Both are fine ARBs. Which one do you think the physician will grab? If it's me, I try to get rid of the excess Diovan. Knowing this tendency, drug reps try to leave as many sample boxes as the office staff will tolerate.

Even before I outlawed free samples permanently from my office in 2005, my staff and I were refusing them on a daily basis. We just didn't have room. As many as a dozen sales representatives would barrage us with drugs in a single day! If we didn't discourage them, every cabinet, drawer, closet, shelf, and counter in the place would be jam-packed with sample drugs. At a certain point, we couldn't wait to get rid of the stuff. Instead of choosing a new drug based solely on its potential, the selection might be based on how much storage space was freed up by dumping the samples. As anyone who has been the beneficiary in the free-sample scheme will attest, you don't just get a few tablets to try, you get bagfuls. So if you are taking an essential medicine that is among those sampled to your doctor, there may be ample quantities to be had at no cost. Here's how to get them: Just ask. Ask at every visit, "Doc, got any samples of Actos for me today?" "Any Plavix samples?" "Do you have any more Fosamax?" "Any more than just those?" You can even call for more between office visits. Ask the staff to request extra boxes from the company representative and stockpile it for you. Admittedly, this is the weakest of the cost-saving methods, because it is not dependable and it is definitely temporary. Still, you can save a lot of money. I have given away the retail equivalent of hundreds of dollars' worth of drug samples to an individual patient at a single office visit, enough to last several months. As long as the freebies last, there is no cost to you, allowing you time to implement other means of obtaining a costly drug.

Take It to the Bank

- Use any and all other cost-saving methods to reduce prescription costs rather than relying on free-sample giveaways from your doctor's office.
- Consider samples if they can cover an entire course of therapy.
- Consider using free samples temporarily while awaiting activation of a pharmacy, drug company, or government assistance program (CSMs 18 through 20).
- At each office visit ask to receive as many free samples as possible of expensive brand-name drugs you must take.
- Call your doctor's office between visits to request they put aside recently acquired samples for you.
- Ask office staff members to request additional boxes of samples for you when company representatives visit.
- Use one or more of the next three cost-saving methods for a more reliable way to continue to afford essential, irreplaceable treatments.

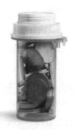

7

Programs for Pills

Cost-Saving Methods 18 through 20

IS YOUR WALLET STILL TOO SMALL to carry the enormous heap of cash you need to bring to the drugstore? Then let me introduce you to cost-saving methods (CSMs) 18,19, and 20. These last three give the inside scoop on getting medicines cheap, *real* cheap. In fact, you might even score some drugs free. Read on and learn how to get some generous breaks from the last ones you'd expect—pharmacies, drug companies, and Uncle Sam himself!

CSM 18: Take Advantage of Giveaways and Discounts

CSM 18 takes advantage of discounts and giveaways for those earning too much to qualify for government assistance. You don't have to be destitute to qualify for these programs; you just have to indicate a need. In some cases even families with considerable assets or higher incomes can meet requirements if medical expenses are eating up too much of the household budget. Before pursuing any of these, however, you should apply the previous CSMs. Why keep jumping through hoops to get costly drugs you don't need or for which there are very affordable substitutions? It is always more satisfying to arrive at a manageable list of drugs than to go begging to the same companies that are gouging you. Moreover, a change in program rules or your financial status could leave you stuck with untenable pharmacy bills once again. If, despite earnestly working through the first seventeen CSMs, you are still left with an expensive treatment regimen, this would be your next step.

Drug Companies with a Heart

Few patients or doctors realize that most drug companies have programs providing prescription drugs *at no cost* to those who can least afford them. In 2006, GlaxoSmithKline gave free prescriptions worth $370 million to more than 400,000 patients.[1] Merck provided nearly 7 million free prescriptions the year prior.[2] Abbott granted over $235 million in savings to over 200,000 patients without drug coverage that year.[3] At least 180 manufacturers have patient-assistance programs, giving away more than 2,500 different medicines. In 2004, over 22 million free prescriptions were filled, worth an estimated $4 billion.[4] Not too bad, especially considering that these programs are little publicized. Still, countless more could benefit by using them. How can you get in on it? All you need to do is apply.

Eligibility requirements for assistance programs vary among the companies (which can be somewhat secretive about the selection criteria), but even families earning up to $70,000 per year can qualify. Acceptance is often based on income without consideration of assets (not so with government programs), so retirees with a small pension but healthy savings are ideal candidates. In determining qualifying income, medical expenses may be subtracted, enabling even those with higher incomes to qualify. What's more, pharmaceutical representatives have told me that administrators do not always ask for proof of income; they'll sometimes take your word for it. So don't assume anything about your eligibility. You won't know until you apply. Those who qualify are typically folks who don't have prescription drug coverage and earn too much to get government assistance. Patients whose prescription costs exceed their annual insurance limits may also qualify.

To take advantage of the pharmaceutical giveaway, the first thing to do is to find out who makes the expensive drugs you take. Usually, the name of the manufacturer is written right on the prescription bottle. If you can't figure it out, your pharmacist or doctor can certainly help you. The *Physician's Desk Reference* (PDR) lists all patented drugs by manufacturer. Once you identify the manufacturer, give them a call. Toll-free directory assistance (1-800-555-1212) has the number. If you are Internet savvy, check drug-company websites, which usually have a link for assistance programs from which you can download or request application forms by mail.

The application process, which can be extensive, will vary by company, and admission criteria change frequently. Your doctor's office may also need to file paperwork or call for approval. If you meet with resistance from your doctor's office staff, explain that in order for you to enroll in the free-drug program the doctor must take part, but that you will pay the usual office fees for filling out forms. If the staff is still uncooperative, schedule an appointment to discuss the application process with your doctor and bring all forms with you. Most doctors will try to help. Upon approval, you may be directed to get your first month's prescription from a local pharmacy using coupons requiring a co-payment. Thereafter, the manufacturer will mail the medication either directly to you or to your doctor's office for dispensing. In some cases you will receive a pharmacy card that allows prescriptions to be filled free of charge at local drugstores. Enrollment renewal is periodically required.

Acquisitions, mergers, reorganizations, bankruptcies, and other corporate shenanigans result in varying requirements and inconstant names for these programs. Some names include "Connection to Care" (Pfizer), "Bridges to Access" (GlaxoSmithKline), and "Access to Medicines" (Lilly).

The sheer number of programs makes it difficult to generalize about eligibility requirements, the application process, and medication procurement methods. Some companies even admit to making approvals on a case-by-case basis. The important message is that these programs are out there, you may very well qualify, and the medicine is free. All you have to do is apply.

Advocacy Is the Best Medicine

There are also patient advocacy groups such as the Free Medicine Foundation, Indigent Patient Services, Inc., and the Medicine Bridge that will go through the application process for you. They charge a set fee and/or per-drug amount to do what you can do yourself, but the cost is nominal considering how tedious the application process can be. They will also process separate applications for each of the expensive drugs you take. One particularly earnest organization is the Free Medicine Program (1-800-921-0072 or www.freemedicine. com). Established by volunteers, they ask only for a one-time fee of $5 that can be refunded if they don't get you your medicines for free. Avoid patient advocacy groups that have *ongoing* monthly charges.

One of the best vehicles I have seen for accessing prescription assistance programs is the Partnership for Prescription Assistance (PPA Rx, at 1-888-4PPA-NOW or www.pparx.org). This industry-sponsored organization offers a single point of access to more than 475 public and private patient-assistance programs, including more than 150 programs offered by pharmaceutical companies. Its website is particularly useful in matching your specific treatments with one or more programs for which you qualify. You simply choose the drugs you are taking from an alphabetized list and answer several inquiries regarding age, state of residence, income, and insurance status. You are then linked to the programs for which you qualify and can download or request applications by mail.

Since the advent of the new Medicare prescription benefit program, many (but not all) private-company assistance programs have dried up for Medicare-eligible patients. Be warned that PPA Rx tries to steer Medicare patients toward Medicare Part D at every opportunity. Although this will usually be profitable for the drug companies (funding expensive drug purchases with tax dollars), it is not necessarily *your* best cost-saving option (see CSM 20).

Drug Companies with a Discount

Many pharmaceutical companies also offer discount cards for those with limited income. Approved drugs can be purchased at savings of 15 to 40 percent or with a nominal co-payment. Most cards are specific to one company, but the Together Rx Access card covers 275 brand-name medicines (and other prescription products) as well as a range of generic drugs from a group of manufacturers. Abbott Laboratories, AstraZenica, Bristol-Meyers Squibb, GlaxoSmithKline, Janssen Pharmaceutica, Ortho McNeil, Novartis, Pfizer, Sanofi-Aventis, Takeda Pharmaceuticals, Tap Pharmaceutical Products, and subsidiaries of Johnson & Johnson are the participating companies. Eligibility requires US citizenship, *ineligibility* for Medicare, no current prescription drug coverage, and income ranging below $30,000 per year for an individual and up to $70,000 for a family of five. Covered drugs can be purchased at up to 40 percent discounts. Savings depend on the particular drug, the quantity, and pharmacy where purchased. Applications are available at pharmacies, doctors' offices, or by calling 1-800-444-4106.

In addition to their free-giveaway program, Merck offers two discount programs to those without health insurance, regardless of age. There is a 10 percent instant-savings certificate that can be printed from their website (www.merck.com/merckhelps/uninsured/home.html) and a Merck Prescription Discount Program Card (which requires completion of an enrollment form) offering 15 to 40 percent savings on a few of their most popular products. You can apply by visiting the above website or calling at 1-908-423-1000. Other companies also offer discounts. It never hurts to contact a manufacturer of your expensive drugs and find out what is available.

Pharmacy Discount Cards

Pharmacy benefit managers (PBMs) such as Caremark also offer discount cards for uninsured or underinsured cash-paying patients. One such card is called RxSavings Plus. The card is accepted at over fifty-seven thousand pharmacies nationwide, providing an average savings of 20 percent off the regular retail price. There are no exclusions or restrictions as long as your purchase is not covered by insurance. RxSavings Plus offers an even higher percentage of savings on selected medications and on three-month supplies ordered by mail through Caremark's mail-service pharmacy. You can enroll online at www.rxsavingsplus.com or call 1-877-673-3688.

Mail-Order Discounts

Outreach Rx is a patient assistance program offered by the mail-order pharmacy Express Scripts (another PBM). This program is available to individuals of all ages with incomes of up to two-and-a-half times the federal poverty level (about $50,000 per year for a family of four). There is no cost to join, just a $20 or $30 co-payment for each prescription for up to a three-month supply of medicine ordered by mail. There is a simple annual enrollment form you can download and print at www.rxoutreach.com (or call for one at 1-800-769-3880). Then just mail your doctor's written prescription with the co-payment to Rx Outreach, Express Scripts Specialty Distribution Services, Inc., PO Box 66536, St. Louis, MO 63166-6536. Medication will be sent directly to you by mail. The formulary of available drugs is somewhat limited, and some of the generic drugs can be purchased at a local pharmacy for cheaper than the co-payment! Still, for many medications, a substantial savings can be realized for a minimal effort.

Where There's a Plan, There's a Scam

There are now health discount cards offered by the hundreds, offering not only discounts on prescriptions, but also medical, dental, hospital, and vision care. These are membership organizations that pool buying power to allow savings on health care products and services. Most are run by private, for-profit businesses. Unlike health insurance, discount cards are not regulated, and that invites scams and chicanery. Watch out for any claims, false "seals of approval," or other suggestions that seem to say a discount card is sponsored by a government agency or a well-known organization. Be wary of discount cards that require you to pay large sums in advance. The fees for most legitimate discount cards are usually fairly low, under $5 for a membership, and perhaps an administration fee. (Some marketing companies take an existing card, package it under a new name, and charge double for the new card!) Ask your doctor, local hospital, pharmacy, and other providers if they accept a card before you sign up, and always check the card's refund policy. You should always have the option to cancel at any time and receive a refund.

It is not only smaller, fly-by-night operations that are implicated in fraudulent pharmacy discount practices. Even the country's largest pharmacy benefit managers, Medco, Caremark, and Express Scripts, have come under scrutiny by prosecutors and consumer advocates for fraud, price-gouging, and violations of standard consumer protection practices.[5] When subscribing to any PBM-administered plan, be watchful of prescription delays, cancellations, and unauthorized or unwanted substitutions. Always make sure you receive the total quantity you have paid for and the specific medicine you and your doctor have agreed upon.

Take It to the Bank

- Most drug companies have programs providing prescription drugs at no cost to those who can least afford them. Find out who makes the expensive drugs you take and call for an application.
- Patient-advocacy groups can go through the application process for you for a nominal fee.

- The Partnership for Prescription Assistance (1-888-4PPA-NOW or www.pparx.org) provides a single point of access to more than 475 public and private patient-assistance programs, including more than 150 programs offered by pharmaceutical companies.
- Many pharmaceutical companies offer discount cards for those with limited income. Call to apply.
- Pharmacy benefit managers (PBMs) such as Caremark and Express Scripts also offer discount mail-order programs and discount cards for uninsured or underinsured cash-paying patients. (See warnings on previous page.)

CSM 19: Uncle Sam Wants You (to Get Your Medicines Cheap)

The only thing better than getting your prescriptions cheap is having someone else pay for them. Sure, you want to eliminate the drugs you don't need or that don't work (CSMs 1 through 4), and no one should take a drug when a change in lifestyle or a nondrug therapy would work better (CSMs 5 through 7). But when taking medication is the best option, have somebody else pick up the tab. Uncle Sam is just the guy.

In no way am I suggesting that you should cheat the system or shirk your responsibility to pay your own way. However, if you have served honorably in the US military, or are dependent on someone who has, you have the right and privilege to receive this benefit. Those with limited income may also be eligible for prescription benefits under Medicaid or with Medicare Part D's Extra Help. Read on to discover programs in which the federal or state government pays for most or all of your prescriptions.

Veterans Affairs (VA)

This is one of the highest-impact yet most underutilized cost-saving programs. If you've had an honorable discharge from the US armed services and need help obtaining essential medicines, fortune has just smiled on you! Enrollment in the VA Health Care System should enable you to get most or all of your medicines for a nominal co-payment ($8 per prescription per month in 2008) or possibly free.

The US Department of Veterans Affairs (VA) provides a medical benefits package including prescription and over-the-counter medication benefits. Officially, only veterans with special eligibility may receive medications prescribed by a non-VA provider. But in practice, VA providers will repre-scribe any medications on the VA formulary (approved list of drugs) that you are already taking. Your outpatient evaluation is often provided by a physician's assistant or nurse practi-tioner. These providers usually won't overrule your private doctors's treatment recommendations and will continue your same prescriptions as long as they are on the VA formulary. Although you will need to see the VA practitioner periodically, nobody expects you to abandon your personal doctor or spe-cialists. In my experience, the VA clinicians are respectful of and integrate nicely with the private community physicians.

Nowhere has the federal government shown an ability to regulate prescription costs better than within the VA. The VA has a fairly comprehensive formulary and negotiates with pharmaceutical companies for the best prices. They have employed some of the same techniques used in my cost-saving methods, such as splitting higher dose tablets, to further reduce costs. Depending on your status, prescriptions obtained through the VA program from a VA pharmacy will be free or have a nominal co-payment, and even this is waived when a certain annual cap in total medication costs is reached. The only drawback is that not all of the drugs prescribed by your private doctor may be on the VA formulary. In this case, working with your doctors to make careful substitutions as described with CSMs 10, 11, and 12, or applying any other appropriate cost-saving methods may bring prescription costs within your budget.

Eligibility for most veterans' health care benefits is based solely on honorable discharge status following active military service in the Army, Navy, Air Force, Marines, or Coast Guard (or Merchant Marines during World War II). Enrollment requires completion of an application form (10–10ez) available from your local VA office and submission of a copy of your discharge document (DD–214 or equivalent). If a VA medical facility or office cannot be found in your local telephone book, you can also call 1-877-222-VETS toll free for information.

TRICARE (Formerly Champus)

The US Department of Defense offers a health care program including pharmacy benefits for active, reserve, or retired uniformed armed services members and their families called TRICARE. It covers the major military branches, the Coast Guard, the Public Health Service, and the National Oceanic and Atmospheric Administration. Active-duty and retired service members and their spouses, children, and stepchildren are eligible beneficiaries. Active-duty and retired reserve component service members and their families are also eligible. In most cases widows and widowers of active-duty members remain eligible unless they remarry. Dependent parents and parents-in-law may also be eligible for the Senior Pharmacy Program under an aligned program called TRICARE Plus.

Eligible beneficiaries may fill prescription medications at military treatment facility pharmacies at no cost, or through the TRICARE Mail-Order Pharmacy or at TRICARE retail network pharmacies for a $3 to $22 co-payment (for up to a ninety-day supply). Prescriptions filled at nonnetwork pharmacies cost $9 to $22 or a 20 to 50 percent co-payment after a $100 to $300 deductible, depending on your plan. Beneficiaries need a valid Uniformed Services ID card. To verify eligibility, visit the Defense Enrollment Eligibility Reporting System (DEERS) page on the TRICARE website (www.tricare. osd.mil/), or call the Defense Manpower Data Center Support Office (1-800-538-9552).

Medicare-eligible beneficiaries continue to be eligible for TRICARE, including pharmacy benefits, in a program called TRICARE for Life. Begun in 2001, this program requires only modest co-payments (no enrollment fees or premiums) for uniformed services beneficiaries over sixty-five years of age. Co-payments are lower for prescriptions filled through the National Mail Order Program and retail pharmacies that belong to the Department of Defense network. Nonnetwork pharmacies can also be used, although with a higher co-payment and after an annual deductible has been met. Enrollment in Medicare Part B is required unless you were born before April 1, 1936. For more information, call 1-888-DOD-LIFE, or visit the TRICARE website listed above.

CHAMPVA

Families of veterans who have a 100 percent, permanent disability, or of veterans who have died from a service-connected disability, may be covered by CHAMPVA (as long as they are not also eligible for TRICARE). Eligible former spouses who lost their TRICARE eligibility when they remarried and whose marriage ended in divorce or death may also be entitled to CHAMPVA. This program is administered by the Department of Veterans Affairs. Veterans may contact the Department of Veterans Affairs toll-free (1-800-827-1000) for information. Details on CHAMPVA eligibility for family members are available from the Veterans Affairs Health Administration Center (1-800-733-8387).

Extra Help Is There When You Need It

Medicare eligible patients with limited income and assets may qualify for Extra Help, a division of Medicare Part D without the usual premiums and deductibles. Co-payments are only $1 to $5 per prescription. Income criteria vary year to year, but you would be eligible for Extra Help in 2006 if your 2005 income was no more than $14,355 for an individual, or $19,245 for a married couple. Higher-income individuals may also qualify for reduced premiums and a lower deductible. Applications are available through the Social Security

Administration, but you can also apply by phone (1-800-772-1213) or via Internet (www.socialsecurity.gov). If you are already receiving Medicaid, a Medicare Savings Program (which pays your Medicare Part B premium),* or Supplemental Security Income (SSI), you are automatically eligible and should have been assigned to an approved Medicare drug plan.

State Pharmaceutical Assistance Programs

As of January 2006, forty-one states had established or authorized subsidy or discount programs to provide pharmaceutical coverage or assistance to low-income elderly or disabled persons who do not qualify for Medicaid. Eligibility requirements of the state subsidy programs can be found on the National Conference of State Legislatures website (www .ncsl.org/programs/health/drugaid.htm#Subsidy). In several states, discount programs have been added to or integrated with subsidy programs. These are compiled in another table on the same website at www.ncsl.org/programs/health/ drugaid.htm#Discount. Otherwise you can inquire about the existence of such programs in your state by contacting your state's department of health or social services.

Medicaid and Medi-Cal

Medicaid is a federal and state entitlement program providing medical assistance including prescription benefits

---

* Medicare Savings Programs such as the Qualified Medicare Beneficiary (QMB), the Qualifying Individuals (QI), and the Specified Low-Income Medicare Beneficiary (SLMB) programs pay Medicare premiums and co-pays for some people with limited incomes.

to certain individuals and families with limited income and resources. (Medicaid is called Medi-Cal in California.) Each state sets its own guidelines regarding eligibility and services. Low income is only one test for Medicaid eligibility. Assets, resources, and designation within certain groups ("categorically needy," "medically needy," or "special") will also determine eligibility. The categorically needy include infants, children, and their caretakers; pregnant women; SSI recipients; and individuals and couples who are living in medical institutions. Medically needy include aged, blind, and disabled persons. The special group includes Medicare beneficiaries whose income is at or below the federal poverty level, qualified working disabled individuals, women who have breast or cervical cancer, and patients with tuberculosis. Medicaid provides coverage for most prescription drugs, so if you think your economic status places you anywhere close to qualifying, look into it. Keep in mind that children may qualify even if their parents do not.

Medicare Part D

The Medicare Prescription Drug Improvement and Modernization Act (MMA) of 2003 provides for the largest government-sponsored prescription benefit program in US history. The complexity of this government program has earned it its own section (see CSM 20).

Take It to the Bank

- Government programs and entitlements can offer coverage of prescription and nonprescription drugs.

- Many eligible veterans are not taking advantage of their health care benefits provided by the US Department of Veterans Affairs, which include coverage of prescription and over-the-counter drugs.

- The US Department of Defense offers a health care program including pharmacy benefits for active, reserve, or retired uniformed armed-services members and their families called TRICARE.

- Dependent parents and parents-in-law may also be eligible for the Senior Pharmacy Program under an aligned program called TRICARE Plus.

- Medicare-eligible beneficiaries continue to be eligible for TRICARE including pharmacy benefits in a program called TRICARE for Life.

- Families of veterans who have a 100 percent, permanent disability, or of veterans who died from a service-connected disability, may be covered by CHAMPVA.

- Medicare eligible patients with limited income and assets may qualify for Extra Help, a division of Medicare Part D without the usual premiums and deductibles.

- Forty-one of the fifty states have established or authorized subsidy or discount programs to provide pharmaceutical coverage or assistance to low-income elderly or disabled persons who do not qualify for Medicaid.

- Medicaid is a federal and state entitlement program providing medical assistance including prescription benefits to certain individuals and families with limited income and resources.

CSM 20: Join Medicare Part D?

Signing up for Medicare Part D, the government prescription drug benefit plan, should be the *last* thing you do. I don't mean to say that enrolling in the plan couldn't save you money or that no one should do it. That's ridiculous; it's one of my cost-saving methods after all. But it should be the final method. All other means described in this book should be employed first. After everything possible has been done to lower your prescription costs, including using discount retailers, you should then assess the benefits of joining.

You could sign up right off and save some money on your current, expensive prescriptions. Perhaps you've already done so. But you'll save more by using as many of the other cost-saving methods as possible first. It may be cheaper to just buy a refined medication regimen (at discount prices!) than to pay the deductibles, premiums, and co-payments required by a benefit plan. Still, you cannot be certain of any advantage until you have brought drug treatment costs under control. If you do stand to benefit by enrolling, you won't be able to choose the plan best suited to match your treatments until your most cost-effective regimen has been determined.

Consider the case of Fanny, a seventy-five-year-old woman taking Diovan for blood pressure and Januvia for diabetes at a yearly cost of $2,586. Her savings under the standard benefit Medicare prescription drug plan would be $1,373.25 (see table 7-1). That sounds pretty good, but if we just apply CSM 12 (using a cheaper class of medicine for the same treatment goal), Fanny's annual pharmacy bill reduces to under $70!

That's a savings of over $2,500, without the headaches of dealing with a prescription plan (table 7-2).

Keep in mind that Medicare prescription drug plans are also insurance policies. The idea is to hedge against catastrophic prescription costs in years to come. As with most insurance, getting coverage early ensures a lower premium. Unlike most insurance, you cannot be denied coverage at your time of need (but you may have to wait several months until

TABLE 7-1: Fanny's Savings with Medicare D Standard Benefit	
1 year of premiums at $30/mo.	$360
Deductible	$275
25% co-pay [0.25 x ($2586 - $275)]	$577.75
Yearly cost	$1,212.75
Yearly savings ($2,586 - $1,254):	**$1,373.25**

TABLE 7-2: Fanny's Savings with Cost-Saving Method 12		
Before		
DRUG	**DOSE**	**COST***
Diovan	80 mg, 1 daily	$720
Januvia	100 mg, 1 daily	$1,866
TOTAL		**$2,586**
After		
DRUG	**DOSE**	**COST***
HCTZ	25 mg, $1/2$ daily	$24
Glipizide	10 mg, 1 daily	$44
TOTAL		**$68**
Yearly Savings ($2586 - $68):		**$2,518**

* Average retail price for one year's supply.

the next enrollment period). The penalty for delaying enrollment is a premium increase of 1 percent of the national average for every month past eligibility. If you become eligible at age sixty-five but don't enroll until age seventy (assuming a national premium average of $55 per month at that time), you would pay a monthly premium surcharge of $33. (Of course, the premiums you didn't pay for the previous five years could cover six to seven years of surcharges.) For many people with nominal prescription costs—or people who bring costs under control with my program—a low premium plan makes the most sense. Others may want to postpone joining until they need coverage.

The Medicare prescription drug benefit is offered through stand-alone prescription drug plans (PDPs) and through Medicare Advantage plans: HMOs, and PPOs that combine supplemental medical insurance (for the 20 percent not covered by Medicare) with a prescription drug benefit. Eligible enrollees in most states have fifty or more stand-alone PDPs to choose from.

Who Can Sign Up

You can only enroll in Medicare Part D if you are eligible for Medicare. Those with both Medicare and Medicaid (or Medi-Cal, in California) are automatically enrolled, and will not have a monthly premium or secondary deductible. Essentially, you are eligible for Medicare if the following apply to you:

- You are sixty-five or older, you are a citizen or permanent resident of the United States, and you or your spouse worked in Medicare-covered employment for at least ten years.

- You are under age sixty-five with a disability or with permanent kidney failure requiring dialysis or transplant.

To apply for Medicare, call the Social Security Administration toll-free number (1-800-772-1213), visit your local Social Security office, or apply online at www.medicare.gov.

The annual open-enrollment period for Medicare Part D is from November 15 to December 31. You can enroll outside the enrollment period if you are newly eligible (the three months before or after your sixty-fifth birthday).

Who Should Sign Up

It's quite simple: unless you are just buying future prescription insurance, you should sign up for Medicare Part D if it will save you money. Determining *whether* it will save you money is the complicated part. (I blame Congress.) But first you must use the other cost-saving methods to arrive at the lowest practical prescription cost. A Kaiser Family Foundation study estimated that about one in four seniors already pays less for drugs than the cost of a typical PDP. With the cost-saving methods, many more people can get below this threshold. When you consider that about half of the top-thirty most-prescribed drugs can be purchased for less than $15 a month, it seems reasonable that many more seniors could work with their doctors to keep prescription costs below the price of prescription insurance.

Congress originally drew up a model plan called the Defined Standard Benefit, but 90 percent of PDPs have their own designs. There are so many variables among the thousands of PDPs available that determining at what point joining begins to save you money is taxing. But to help you decide if Medicare Part D would be worthwhile, I offer the following general guidelines (applicable to the Defined Standard Benefit at the average national premium rate for 2008):

- For annual prescription costs less than about $750, a PDP would be more expensive than buying your drugs retail.
- For drug costs between $1,000 and $2,500, the savings range from about 20 to 50 percent—definitely worthwhile.
- Drug costs between $2,500 and $5,700 per year are not covered by most PDPs, and available coverage in this range is usually a poor value (see "Secondary Deductibles—the Coverage Gap," page 187).
- Annual prescription costs above $5,700 are 95 percent covered.

What Are the Costs?

There are four categories of costs associated with the Medicare prescription benefit program: premiums, co-payments, primary deductibles, and secondary deductibles (the coverage gap or "doughnut hole"). Some or all of these costs may apply, depending on the plan you choose and the drugs you take.

Premiums

The premium is a monthly fee for participation in a PDP. Across the country, premiums range from about $10 to $110.*

* Prices in 2008.

The average premium is about $30, and 40 percent of plans are priced below that. This average represents a 17 percent increase since 2006. One in four enrollees saw premium increases of 50 percent or more from 2006 to 2008[6]—disturbing trends for those on fixed incomes. If your monthly premium rises, look around for a better deal. There were 249 organizations offering 4,847 different plans in 2007, all vying for your business.[7] Changing plans when premiums rise helps keep rates competitive, yet less than 10 percent of affected enrollees did so in 2007.[8] If your prescription costs are negligible and you are attracted to the idea of securing lower premiums now for possible coverage later, choose a plan with the lowest possible premium. You can change plans to match your needs later without penalty.

The premium may be paid passively (withheld from your Social Security, Railroad Retirement, or Civil Service Retirement check), or sent in monthly. Lower premiums usually mean higher costs in other categories, while higher premiums typically offer more generous benefits.

Primary Deductibles

The primary deductible is a specified amount you must pay for your prescription drugs before the plan pays anything. For 2008 the Defined Standard Benefit drawn up by Congress has a $275 deductible, but less than a third of national PDPs follow this. Ten percent have a lower deductible, and the rest (60 percent) have no deductible.[9] So if avoiding a deductible is your aim, it should be easy to find a plan without this expense.

Co-Payments

A co-payment is the uncovered amount for a prescription purchase—the part of the cost that you must pay. It can vary with the type or quantity of medicine, or with the pharmacy where the drug is purchased. Most PDPs have flat dollar co-payments corresponding to differing groups, or *tiers*, of drugs. Seventy-five percent of these plans have *three* cost-sharing tiers: the first for generic drugs, the second for preferred brand-name drugs, and the third for nonpreferred drugs. The remaining plans have two or four tiers. A new design in 2008 has four tiers, dividing generic drugs further into preferred and nonpreferred types.

In 2008, the average co-payment for the generic tier was about $5 for a thirty-day supply of medication. This may seem like a good deal, but $5 per month is higher than the discount price of some of the most widely prescribed generic drugs. Alprazolam, atenolol, and hydrochlorothiazide are among the top-ten most prescribed drugs, and can each be purchased (in quantity) for less than $5 per month. In addition, some discount retailers sell many popular generic drugs for $4 or $5 for a thirty-day supply. So if all of your drugs are generic, it is probably cheaper to buy them retail than to enroll in the Medicare program with an average of $360 per year in premiums in addition to the $5 per month co-payments.

Preferred tier drugs have an average co-payment of about $30, and nonpreferred tier drugs have an average co-payment of about $70. These are the *average* co-payments. You should shop for PDPs offering lower amounts. Co-payments may be lower for three-month mail-away prescriptions. You also want the preferred tier of your chosen PDP to include the brand-name drugs you can't change. If you are taking several brand-name products, it may require some investigation to find a preferred formulary containing all of them. Some pharmacies will do a search as a free service. Just present them with a list of your medicines and ask which PDP has a preferred tier with them all. Better yet, using the cost-saving methods, you can adapt your drug treatments to generic and preferred tiers of a PDP you can afford.

For the best economy, avoid the nonpreferred tier! Co-payments average $70 but may be as high as $107 for a month of medication. Either choose a PDP where all of your drugs are in lower co-payment tiers, or use CSMs 10 through 12 to adjust your regimen to consist only of medicines in the generic and preferred tiers.

To confound things more, most plans now have a *specialty* tier for the most expensive drugs. Medicare guidelines limit the co-payment for these purchases to 33 percent of the prescription cost. As much as possible, use the CSMs to avoid drugs from this tier since the out-of-pocket costs can be painful.

Co-payments may also be based on a *percentage* of the prescription cost, in which case tiers are not used. The percentage varies with the total amount of prescription expenditure for the year. This is the case for the standard benefit drawn up by Congress. The co-payment is 25 percent for the first $2,500 in drug costs (after meeting the $275 deductible), and 5 percent after total pharmacy costs reach about $5,700. (Between $2,500 and $5,700 is the coverage gap.) Although this was the scheme Congress envisioned for the prescription benefit, 90 percent of PDPs use tiered flat-dollar co-payments instead.

Secondary Deductibles—the Coverage Gap

The secondary deductible is a gap in coverage you must pay when drug expenses are more than a certain amount, but less than another designated amount. (Again, I blame Congress.) The gap was included because the cost of providing continuous coverage with no gap would have exceeded the Medicare's drug budget. Continuous coverage might have required Medicare to negotiate with pharmaceutical companies on drug prices, a provision that is expressly prohibited by the Medicare Modernization Act. In 2008, the coverage gap totals $3,216. By 2016, it will exceed $6,000—more bad news for seniors on fixed incomes.[10] Part D enrollees who qualify for Extra Help (the low-income subsidy), or who have Medicare and Medicaid, are not responsible for costs in the gap.

Only 30 percent of PDPs currently offer gap coverage, and all of these (except for one plan in Florida) cover only generic drugs once expenses reach the coverage gap. Of these plans, half only cover *some* generics. Premiums for plans with gap coverage are double those of PDPs without gap coverage, averaging over $63 per month. Unless you are taking half a dozen or more generic drugs (along with the ones putting you into the gap), this is a poor value. The savings on the lower premium PDPs would probably cover the cost of these drug purchases since most generics are reasonably priced. Most seniors have figured this one out, as only a few percent of enrollees choose plans with gap coverage.

Avoid the Gap!

Above $2,500 in annual prescription drug costs, you enter the coverage gap. Beyond this amount, for most plans, the next $3,216 in prescription costs are all yours. Standard PDPs offer little help in this range, although Medicare Advantage insurance plans may have some benefits. This is where the cost-savings methods can really make a difference. Consider the case of Vera, a ninety-two-year-old woman with emphysema, depression, and osteoporosis who was prescribed Duoneb, Advair, Zoloft, and Fosamax. On this regimen, her total yearly prescription tally was $4,640, above the $2,500 mark and well into the uncovered gap. With the standard benefit, her yearly out-of-pocket costs were $3,331 ($1191 [for the first $2500] + $2140 [the uncovered "gap" amount]). Unfortunately, this sum was unaffordable, making the Medicare benefit inadequate for her. But a review of her medications with application of the cost-saving methods allowed us to reduce her total yearly prescription burden to $1,354, which under Medicare Part D cost her $905, within her budget and providing a savings of over $2,400 per year! *

Out of the Hole and Back into the Doughnut

Above $5,700 in yearly prescription costs, the savings with Medicare D become substantial. The model plan covers 95 percent of costs above this amount. Prescription costs of $7,500 per year would cost you $4,481 under the standard

* Vera's medication changes with direct price comparisons are provided in detail on the *How to Save on Prescription Drugs* website, www. howtosaveondrugs.com.

benefit, a savings of about 40 percent. I don't know about you, but I still think the $4,481 you would have to spend is a lot of money. It's better than paying $7,500, of course, but it is still beyond the budget of many seniors. To my way of thinking, this denotes a major flaw in the Medicare drug benefit program. Although the 95 percent coverage of prescription costs above $5,700 seems impressive, to keep total prescription drug costs under the Medicare program reasonable, it is still best to stay under the gap.

How to Find Your Plan

Each PDP specifies its own premium, deductible, gap coverage, and co-payments. Each offers unique lists of approved drugs (the formularies) and utilizes specific pharmacy networks. This many variables make comparisons among the plans tricky—especially if you have fifty or more to choose from. The most practical way to compare all of the available plans in your area is by using the Medicare website (www .medicare.gov). If you don't have Internet access, have someone who does help you. Under "Search Tools" on the home page, click on "Compare Medicare Prescription Drug Plans," and then click on "Find & Compare Plans." The website will guide you through entering your zip code, age, health status, and current coverage. You can then enter your prescription drug names and continue to see a list of all of the plans in your area. The premium, deductible, gap coverage, and estimated annual cost of each plan are listed in table format next to the plan. There are links allowing you to enroll in a selected plan right then and there, with the coverage and out-of-pocket costs plainly indicated.

A plan that serves your neighbor may not be as suitable for you, so you must do your own shopping. But no matter which plan you choose, your cost will always be lower if your prescription costs are lower in general. This is why the cost-saving methods should always be applied even if you are eligible or already enrolled in Medicare part D. In no way should Medicare eligibility be viewed as an excuse for having an overpriced or inflated drug regimen. Inefficient or expensive prescribing will always cost you more.

By law, all plan formularies will have at least two agents per drug class. That leaves out a lot of drugs. Regardless of the cost, it may be hard to find a plan that covers all of your current medicines in its formulary tiers. The more drugs you take, the less likely it will be that one plan's formulary will have them all. Another drug from the same class (as discussed in CSM 11) or from a different class with the same treatment goal may need to be substituted (CSM 12) to fit your treatment to a single PDP. Such exchanges and substitutions should be made one at a time under the careful supervision of your doctor. However, while you will be locked into an individual PDP for a full year, the plan can change the drugs in its formulary monthly! That provision could mean an unrealistic and unhealthy amount of switching drugs. The goal in this game is to find or adapt to a plan that covers all of your drugs, minimizes premiums and co-payments, and permits convenient drug purchases.

If you already have prescription drug coverage under Medicare Advantage, Medigap, your employer, or your union, stick with it. You are probably better off, and there is no penalty for switching from these approved plans to a Medicare PDP later. Drug coverage through the Federal Employees Health Benefits Program (FEHBP) is comparable to Medicare Part D, and there is no penalty for late enrollment as long as you keep coverage. Beneficiaries who are eligible for low-income subsidies (Extra Help) will not have deductibles, but they must complete a five-page application form that includes questions about income and assets.

Take It to the Bank

- To maximize savings, the cost-saving methods should always be applied, even if you are eligible or already enrolled in a Medicare prescription benefit program.
- You can only enroll in Medicare Part D if you are eligible for Medicare.
- You should sign up for Medicare Part D if it will save you money beyond the other cost-saving methods or if you are seeking insurance against future drug needs.
- Forty percent of PDPs have premiums less than $30 per month. The lowest is under $10. Consider changing plans when premiums rise.
- For annual prescription costs less than about $750, a PDP is probably more expensive than buying your drugs retail.

- If your total yearly prescription drug costs are between $1,000 and $2,250, you would save about 20 to 50 percent on your prescriptions by joining the model plan.
- Drug costs between $2,500 and $5,700 per year are not covered by most PDPs, and available coverage in this range is usually a poor value. Use the cost-savings methods to avoid this gap.
- Above $5,700, the model plan covers 95 percent of costs.

A Note on Expiration Dates

You're rummaging through the refrigerator and you discover an unopened container of yogurt, the expensive kind in your favorite flavor. Where did that come from? You haven't bought any yogurt in weeks. But it's just what you were craving. As you struggle with the seemingly impenetrable foil cover, taking care not to splash the thick pink liquid all over yourself, you notice the expiration date stamped on it: that was two weeks ago! What do you do now? Are you the type that just tosses it into the trash, or do you inspect and perhaps taste the contents for freshness first? And, assuming it is still palatable, do you worry that eating it could make you ill?

Similar concerns may cross your mind when you are confronted with the expiration date on a bottle of prescription medicine. Is the medication still potent and effective, or has it degraded into a toxic potion? Does the cost of the medicine influence how willing you are to take pills after the date stamped on the bottle? Should "expired" drugs be flushed into the water supply or donated to the landfill? Millions of dollars of drugs are discarded this way every year. Is this prudent or just a waste of money?

Beyond Use and Still Good

First off, unless you have the actual stock bottle from the manufacturer, the date written on your prescription bottle is not the expiration date at all. That date is the "beyond-use date." In compliance with the standards of the US

Pharmacopoeia (USP), retail pharmacists put this date on the label when they repackage medicine into prescription bottles. The beyond-use date is either one year from the date the prescription is filled or the expiration date on the original manufacturer's container, whichever is sooner. The beyond-use date was increased by the USP in year 2000 from six months to one year.[1] This period of time is a general compromise, since it must apply to so many variables. There are thousands of medications, each with an innate stability. Drugs degrade over time at a huge variation from compound to compound. The stability of any medicine will further vary depending on environmental factors. Who knows how the stuff will be treated after it leaves the pharmacy? Will it be handled, agitated, placed in sunlight, transferred to another container, stored in a cool, dry refrigerator or in a warm, steamy bathroom? What if it freezes? The USP can't know how long it's going to last. Depending on the circumstances, some preparations might degrade before a year after they are dispensed; others could retain potency for decades. But some kind of guidance should be given, so one year is what they've come up with.

There is an expiration date on the manufacturer's packaging, but this is a misnomer. The drug does not "expire" on that date. It is more accurately a "still good" date. It means only that analysis has shown or predicts that the drug will still be stable at that date. After that, no estimate of any decline in potency over time is provided. Once the original container is opened, the expiration date on it no longer applies anyway. Expiration dates for new drugs are usually two to three years beyond the date of manufacture, and therefore may be a year or more later than the beyond-use date on your prescription bottle.

So the manufacturer's expiration dates and pharmacist's "beyond use" dates do not really establish when a loss of potency begins to occur, nor do they tell us how much activity might remain at a given point in time. Pharmaceutical companies don't recommend using medication beyond the expiration date. They would rather have you buy another fresh batch. Because of liability concerns, they don't even comment on the safety and effectiveness of "expired" drugs. Just how long can we expect drugs to retain their potency, then? Well, we can look at what the *Medical Letter on Drugs and Therapeutics* compiled on this topic in 2002.[2]

Drugs That Last

The Department of Defense/FDA Shelf Life Extension Program tested the stability of drugs past their expiration date. Results showed that 84 percent of over one thousand separate lots of about one hundred different drug products (stored in military facilities in their original unopened containers) remained stable for an average of 4.75 years after their original expiration date![3] Stored properly, then, most drugs should retain potency well beyond their expirations dates. Another study looked at the stability of four drugs (Capoten [captopril], Flucloxin [flucloxacillin], Mefoxin [cefoxitin], and Theo-Dur [theophylline]) when stored under conditions of high temperature and humidity. Even when these drugs were stored in 75 percent humidity at 104 degrees Fahrenheit, they remained chemically and physically stable for *up to nine years* beyond their expiration dates.[4] The antiflu drugs amantadine and Flumadine (rimantidine) showed Houdini-like resiliency, remaining stable and retaining full antiviral activity after twenty-five years of storage *and* after being boiled and held at 65 to 85 degrees Centigrade for several days![5] (What kind of person thinks up these experiments, anyway?) Finally, theophylline (Theo-Dur, Theo-24, Uniphyll, and others) has been reported to retain 90 percent of its potency for up to *thirty years* after manufacture.[6] These studies indicate that some drugs remain potent for years beyond their expiration dates, even when stored under adverse conditions.

Let's also alleviate any fears of toxicity caused by a drug that may have chemically changed with time. The only drug ever reported to have done so was some degraded tetracycline back in 1963.[7] (Tetracycline preparations have since been reformulated to prevent degradation.) That's it—no other such toxicities have been reported in humans. So even if you have concerns about the effectiveness of drugs used past their expirations dates, such drugs are unlikely to cause any more adverse affects than they would when fresh out of the factory; the safety is unchanged. With that in mind, then, you could try an expired analgesic for a headache. If the medication is still potent—and it probably is—you may save on an unnecessary trip to the doctor, pharmacy, or emergency room.

The effectiveness of many medications taken past their labeled "beyond-use date" can be easily assessed. Is your blood pressure still just as well controlled? Did the sedative let you fall asleep? Is your heartburn relieved? If the drug still works, potency shouldn't be in question.

Some medications may be taken for indications considered too critical to take any risk of using a batch with reduced potency. Anti-arrhythmia and antiseizure drugs would fall into that category. Also, medicines with a low therapeutic index (see CSM 10), such as levothyroxin, Coumadin (warfarin), and lithium, should not be used if there is any question about the potency or stability of the pills on hand.

Drugs That Don't

What about liquid medicines? How is their stability affected with time? In general, solutions and suspensions are not as stable as solid medications. Certainly you don't want to use any injected medicine, such as insulin, that appears cloudy or discolored, or that has solid particles suspended in it. Oral suspensions and syrups may change color due to degradation of the dyes more than the active ingredients. Drugs suspended in solvents, such as antibiotics for use by mouth, tend to be unstable. Prescription eye drops are prone to bacterial contamination once the added preservatives stop working, so the stability of the actual eye medication may not be as critical as that of the preservative. In general, I would advise against using prescription medicine in liquid form after the beyond-use date, except perhaps for something innocuous such as cough syrup.

Take It to the Bank

- How much potency prescription drugs retain over time varies with the particular medication and the environment in which it is stored. In general, tablets and capsules stored in a cool, dry place (not a steamy shower room!) can be expected to remain potent for years past the expiration date.

- The beyond-use date on the prescription bottle is either the same as the manufacturer's expiration date or, more likely, a year or two sooner.

- There have been no modern reports of toxicity from use of outdated drugs.

- For noncritical conditions requiring expensive drugs, use of medicine after the date on the prescription bottle is safe, is probably just as effective, and can result in considerable savings over repurchase of the medicine.[8]

Afterword: Make This Book Obsolete

In January 2007, I began to speak publicly on saving money on prescription drugs. Auditoriums and parish halls would fill with people anxious to find ways to afford their medicines. The talks were a big success; I could not even schedule all of the groups who wanted to hear my methods on cutting drug costs.

The whole situation was also ridiculous. Only in a system where doctors are oblivious to treatment costs, and where patients passively accept exorbitant therapies, could such lectures be in demand. If doctors knew how to prescribe within patients' budgets, and patients refused to accept otherwise, we all could have stayed home on Sunday nights. Instead, I lectured. Since I did not directly change anyone's treatment myself, what did my audiences get for their time? What tricks did I reveal?

I empowered them to confront their doctors.

Commercial influence might have a big impact on physician prescribing, but it is not as strong as your influence. Do not underestimate the tenacity of the doctor-patient relationship; it is fundamental to the healing arts. You have more power to affect your physician than anyone else (including Pfizer). By improving communication, my audiences learned how to bring economy to their doctors' treatment choices. Your doctor, too, will take cost into consideration if you make it a priority. This is my single best cost-saving method: foster a partnership with your doctor to treat effectively and affordably. Once these ideals are put into practice, we can reclaim faith in the medical profession and improve the quality of health care for all. We can make this book obsolete.

Appendix: Expensive-Drug Survival Index

THE EXPENSIVE-DRUG SURVIVAL INDEX contains an alphabetical listing of the most popular medications costing more than $30 per month at usual doses. Next to each drug is at least one tip that might be used to lower treatment costs. The tips correspond to cost-saving methods 10 through 13, discussed in chapters 5 and 6. Please refer to those chapters for a complete explanation.

The first column contains a "G" when there is a generic equivalent available at a lower price (see CSM 10) and an "S" when the listed medication comes in a tablet form that is suitable for splitting as a cost-saving measure (see CSM 13).

The second column lists cheaper medications from the same family or class (see CSM 11).

The third column contains cheaper medications from alternate classes used for the same purpose (see CSM 12). Where more than one class is represented, they are numbered in no particular order. For columns two and three, not all possible substitutions are listed—only a representative few. Suggested substitutions are either less than $30 per month of treatment at usual doses, or they are significantly cheaper than the listed drug. Note: a plus sign (+) signifies that the two medications should be taken together.

Where more than one cost-saving method is provided, all of the methods may not be simultaneously applicable or bring about the same degree of savings. For example, a same-family substitution may be a better value than splitting a very expensive tablet, even though both possibilities are listed.

The suggested substitutions are not a treatment recommendation for any medical condition. They are simply suggestions that you might discuss with your doctor. No changes in treatment should be made unless under the direct guidance of a treating physician.

Prices of all of the drugs in this table can be checked easily online on CVS.com, Drugstore.com, or FamilyMeds.com. Be sure to bring the cost comparison for any proposed substitution to your doctor for review.

The latest version of the Expensive-Drug Survival Index, with updates on generic availability and class substitutions, is always available on the website www.howtosaveondrugs.com.

EXPENSIVE-DRUG SURVIVAL INDEX			
Drug	**G*** **S****	**Same-class substitutions**	**Alternate-class substitutions**
Abilify	S		1) fluphenazine, haloperidol, thioridazine, thiothixene 2) lithium 3) carbamazepine
Accolate			1) albuterol inhaler 2) beclomethasone inhaler 3) theophylline
Accupril	G S	lisinopril, enalapril, captopril	
Accuretic	G S	lisinopril/HCT, enalapril/ HCT, captopril/HCT	

Drug	G* S**	Same-class substitutions	Alternate-class substitutions
Aceon	S	lisinopril, enalapril, captopril	
Aciphex		omeprazole	1) ranitidine, famotidine 2) OTC antacids
Actonel		alendronate	1) estrogen 2) calcium/vitamin D 3) exercise
Actos Actoplus Met	S		1) glipizide, glyburide 2) metformin
Acular			Advanced Eye Relief, Naphcon-A, Rite Aid Eye Allergy, Visine-A
Adalat CC	G		
Adderall	G S	dextroamphetamine, methylphenidate	
Adderall XR		dextroamphetamine CR, methylphenidate	
Advair Discus		[(albuterol or metaproterenol inhaler) + beclomethasone inhaler]	theophylline
Advicor		lovastatin, pravastatin, simvastatin	
Aerobid		beclomethasone inhaler	
Aggrenox		aspirin + dipyridamole	
Allegra	G	loratidine, cetirizine	cromolyn sodium nasal spray
Altace	S	lisinopril, enalapril, captopril	

*G = generic availability   **S = tablet suitable for splitting

Drug	G* S**	Same-class substitutions	Alternate-class substitutions
Altocor Altoprev	G	lovastatin, pravastatin, simvastatin	
Ambien	G S		1) lorazepam, oxazepam, temazepam 2) trazodone (nonhabit-forming)
Ambien CR		Zolpedem immediate release	1) lorazepam, oxazepam, temazepam 2) trazodone (nonhabit-forming)
Amerge			1) aspirin, naproxen, ketoprofen 2) codeine, hydrocodone 3) prochlorperazine, promethazine 4) ergotamine tartrate 5) isometheptene/acetaminophen 6) butalbital-APAP-caffeine
Arthrotec		[misoprostol + (dicolfenac, ibuprofen, or naproxen)], choline magnesium trisalicylate	
Astelin		loratidine, cetirizine	cromolyn sodium nasal spray

Drug	G* S**	Same-class substitutions	Alternate-class substitutions
Atacand Atacand/HCT	S		1) hydrochlorothiazide, chlorthalidone 2) atenolol, nadolol, propranolol 3) lisinopril, enalapril, captopril 4) diltiazem, verapamil, nifedipine ER 5) clonidine, guanfacine
Avapro	S		1) hydrochlorothiazide, chlorthalidone 2) atenolol, nadolol, propranolol 3) lisinopril, enalapril, captopril 4) diltiazem, verapamil, nifedipine ER 5) clonidine, guanfacine
Avalide			1) atenolol, nadolol, propanolol 2) lisinopril, enalapril, captopril 3) diltiazem, verapamil, nifedipine ER 4) clonidine, guanfacine + hydrochlorothiazide
Avandia, Avandamet Avandaryl	S		1) glipizide, glyburide, glimepiride 2) metformin
Avodart		finasteride	doxazosin, terazosin

*G = generic availability   **S = tablet suitable for splitting

Drug	G* S**	Same-class substitutions	Alternate-class substitutions
Axert	S		1) aspirin, naproxen, ketoprofen 2) codeine, hydrocodone 3) prochlorperazine, promethazine 4) ergotamine tartrate 5) isometheptene/ acetaminophen 6) butalbital-APAP-caffeine
Axid	G	ranitidine	OTC antacids
Azopt			1) timolol, levobunolol 2) brimonidine 3) pilocarpine
Beconase AQ		flunisolide nasal spray	1) loratidine, cetirizine 2) cromolyn sodium nasal spray
Benicar Benicar/HCT	S		1) hydrochlorothiazide, chlorthalidone 2) atenolol, nadolol, propranolol 3) lisinopril, enalapril, captopril 4) diltiazem, verapamil, nifedipine ER 5) clonidine, guanfacine
Betapace	G S		
Boniva		alendronate	1) estrogen 2) calcium/vitamin D 3) exercise
Budeprion	G		fluoxetine, paroxetine, sertraline

Drug	G* S**	Same-class substitutions	Alternate-class substitutions
Buspar	G S		
Byetta			1) glipizide, glyburide, glimepiride 2) metformin 3) insulin
Caduet		[nifedipine ER, felodipine] + [lovastatin, pravastatin, simvastatin]	1) hydrochlorothiazide, chlorthalidone 2) atenolol, nadolol, propranolol 3) lisinopril, enalapril, captopril 4) diltiazem, verapamil, nifedipine ER 5) clonidine, guanfacine + [lovastatin, pravastatin, simvastatin]
Calan, Calan SR	G		
Cardizem CD Cardizem LA	G		
Cardura	G S		
Cataflam	G		
Catapress	G S		
Celebrex		ibuprofen, naproxen, choline magnesium trisalicylate	1) tylenol 2) propoxyphene, codeine, tramadol
Celexa	G S		
Cenestin		estradiol, estropipate	
Cialis	S		
Clarinex Clarinex-D		loratidine, cetirizine	cromolyn sodium nasal spray

*G = generic availability   **S = tablet suitable for splitting

Drug	G* S**	Same-class substitutions	Alternate-class substitutions
Cleocin-T	G		
Climara		estradiol, estropipate	
Combivent		albuterol inhaler, metaproterenol inhaler	
Concerta		dextroamphetamine CR, methylphenidate	
Cordarone	G		
Coreg	G S		
Coreg CR		carvedilol immediate release	
Corgard	G S		
Cosopt		timolol + dorzolamide	brimonidine
Covera HS	G	verapamil CR	
Cozaar	S		1) hydrochlorothiazide, chlorthalidone 2) atenolol, nadolol, propranolol 3) lisinopril, enalapril, captopril 4) diltiazem, verapamil, nifedipine ER 5) clonidine, guanfacine
Crestor	S	lovastatin, pravastatin, simvastatin	
Cymbalta		venlafaxine immediate release	fluoxetine, paroxetine, sertraline
Cytotec	G S		famotidine, ranitidine, nizatidine
Darvocet	G S		
Daypro	G	ibuprofen, naproxen	

Drug	G* S**	Same-class substitutions	Alternate-class substitutions
Daytrana		dextroamphetamine CR, methylphenidate	
Depakene	G		
Desyrel	G S		
Detrol	S	oxybutinin	amitriptyline, doxepin, nortriptyline
Detrol LA		oxybutinin	amitriptyline, doxepin, nortriptyline
Diabeta	G S		
Dilacor XR	G	diltiazem ER	
Diovan Diovan HCT			1) hydrochlorothiazide, chlorthalidone 2) atenolol, nadolol, propranolol 3) lisinopril, enalapril, captopril 4) diltiazem, verapamil, nifedipine ER 5) clonidine, guanfacine
Ditropan	G		
Ditropan XL		oxybutinin immediate release	
Doral	S	lorazepam, temazepam	zolpedem
Doryx	G	doxycycline	
Effexor XR	G	venlafaxine immediate release	fluoxetine, paroxetine, sertraline
Enablex	S	oxybutinin	amitriptyline, doxepin, nortriptyline
Enjuvia	S	estradiol, estropipate	

*G = generic availability   **S = tablet suitable for splitting

Drug	G* S**	Same-class substitutions	Alternate-class substitutions
Estrace	G S		
Estring		estradiol, estropipate	
Etodolac CR		etodolac immediate release	
Evista			1) estrogen 2) alendronate 3) calcium/vitamin D 4) exercise
Exubera		regular insulin	
Famvir	G S	acyclovir	
Fenofibrate		gemfibrozil	lovastatin, pravastatin
Femring		estradiol, estropipate	
Fioricet Fiorinol	G		
Flexeril	G S		
Flomax		doxazosin, terazosin	
Flonase	G	flunisolide	1) loratidine, cetirizine 2) cromolyn sodium nasal spray
Flovent HFA		beclomethasone inhaler	
Focalin XR		dextroamphetamine LA, Focalin IR	
Fortamet		metformin immediate release	
Forteo			1) estrogen 2) alendronate 3) calcium/vitamin D 4) exercise

Drug	G* S**	Same-class substitutions	Alternate-class substitutions
Fosamax	G S		1) estrogen 2) calcium/vitamin D 3) exercise
Fosinopril		lisinopril, enalapril, captopril	
Frova			1) aspirin, naproxen, ketoprofen 2) codeine, hydrocodone 3) prochlorperazine, promethazine 4) ergotamine tartrate 5) isometheptene/acetaminophen 6) butalbital-APAP-caffeine
gabapentin	S		
Geodon			1) fluphenazine, haloperidol, thioridazine, thiothixene 2) lithium 3) carbamazepine
glimepiride	S		
Glucophage	G S		
Glumetza	G	metformin immediate release	
Glynase	G S	nonmicronized glyburide, glipizide, glimepiride	
Glyset	S		1) glipizide, glyburide, glimepiride 2) metformin
Guanabenz	S	clonididne	

*G = generic availability   **S = tablet suitable for splitting

Drug	G* S**	Same-class substitutions	Alternate-class substitutions
Hyzaar	S		1) atenolol, nadolol, propanolol 2) lisinopril, enalapril, captopril 3) diltiazem, verapamil, nifedipine ER 4) clonidine, guanfacine + hydrochlorothiazide
Imdur	G S		
Imitrex	S		1) aspirin, naproxen, ketoprofen 2) codeine, hydrocodone 3) prochlorperazine, promethazine 4) ergotamine tartrate 5) isometheptene/ acetaminophen 6) butalbital-APAP-caffeine
Inspra	S	spironolactone, amelioride, triamterine	
Invega			1) fluphenazine, haloperidol, thioridazine, thiothixene 2) lithium 3) carbamazepine
Iopidine		brimonidine	1) timolol, levobunolol 2) pilocarpine
Ismo	G S		
Isoptin SR	G		
Janumet		metformin + alternate class	glipizide, glyburide, glimepiride

Drug	G* S**	Same-class substitutions	Alternate-class substitutions
Januvia			1) glipizide, glyburide, glimepiride 2) metformin
K-Lor K-Lyte K-Tabs Kaon Kay Ciel	G S	potassium 10 percent liquid, Klor-con	
Kerlone	G	atenolol, propranolol	
Ketoprofen CR		ketoprofen immediate release	
Klonapin	G S		
Lamisil		For toenail fungus: weekly fluconazole	
Lantus		lente insulin, NPH insulin	
Lescol Lescol XL		lovastatin, pravastatin, simvastatin	
Levatol		atenolol, propranolol	
Levimir		lente insulin, NPH insulin	
Levitra	S		
Lexapro	S	citalopram, fluoxetine, paroxetine, sertraline	
Lexxel	G	ACE inhibitor + Ca channel blocker	1) hydrochlorothiazide, chlorthalidone 2) atenolol, nadolol, propranolol 3) clonidine, guanfacine
Lipitor	S	lovastatin, pravastatin, simvastatin	

*G = generic availability   **S = tablet suitable for splitting

Drug	G* S**	Same-class substitutions	Alternate-class substitutions
Lithobid	G	lithium carbonate controlled-release tabs	
Lopid	G		
Lopressor	G		
Lotrel		ACE inhibitor + Ca channel blocker	1) hydrochlorothiazide, chlorthalidone 2) atenolol, nadolol, propranolol 3) clonidine, guanfacine
Lotronex			1) fiber supplements 2) dicyclomine, hyocyamin 3) diphenoxylate, loperamide 4) amitriptyline, imipramine
Lovaza		USP-verified fish-oil capsules	gemfibrozil
Lozol	G		
Lufyllin	S	theophylline	
Lumigan			1) timolol, levobunolol 2) brimonidine 3) pilocarpine
Lunesta	S	zolpedem immediate release	lorazepam, oxazepam, temazepam
Lyrica		gabapentin	amitriptyline, desipramine, doxepin
Mavik	G S	lisinopril, enalapril, captopril	

Drug	G* S**	Same-class substitutions	Alternate-class substitutions
Maxair		albuterol inhaler, metaproterenol inhaler	
Maxalt Maxalt MLT	S		1) aspirin, naproxen, ketoprofen 2) codeine, hydrocodone 3) prochlorperazine, promethazine 4) ergotamine tartrate 5) isometheptene/ acetaminophen 6) butalbital-APAP-caffeine
Menest	S	estradiol, estropipate	
Menostar		estradiol, estropipate	
meprobamate	S	lorazepam, alprazolam	
Metaglip	G	[metformin + (glipizide, glyburide, or glimepiride)]	
metolazone	S	hydrochlorothiazide, chlorthalidone	
Mevacor	G S		
Mexitil	G		
Miacalcin			1) estrogen 2) alendronate 3) calcium/vitamin D 4) exercise

*G = generic availability   **S = tablet suitable for splitting

Drug	G* S**	Same-class substitutions	Alternate-class substitutions
Micardis Micardis HCT	S		1) hydrochlorothiazide, chlorthalidone 2) atenolol, nadolol, propranolol 3) lisinopril, enalapril, captopril 4) diltiazem, verapamil, nifedipine ER 5) clonidine, guanfacine
Micronase	G S		
Miltown	G	alprazolam, lorazepam	
Minocin	G	doxycycline, tetracycline	
Mirapex	S	For RLS: carbidopa/levodopa	For RLS: 1) propoxyphene, hydrocodone 2) clonazepam, oxazepam, zolpidem 3) gabapentin
Mobic	G S	ibuprofen, naproxen	
Monopril	G S	lisinopril, enalapril, captopril	
Nabumetone		ibuprofen, naproxen	
Namenda	S		
Naprelan Naproxen DR	G	naproxen immediate release	
Naprosyn	G		
Nasacort Aq		flunisolide, fluticasone	1) loratidine, cetirizine 2) cromolyn sodium nasal spray
Nasarel	G		1) loratidine, cetirizine 2) cromolyn sodium nasal spray

Drug	G* S**	Same-class substitutions	Alternate-class substitutions
Nasonex		flunisolide, fluticasone	
Neurontin	G S		
Nexium		omeprazole	1) ranitidine, famotidine 2) OTC antacids
Niaspan			lovastatin, pravastatin, simvastatin
Nitro-Dur		isosorbide mononitrate CR	
Nizatidine		ranitidine	
Nolvadex	G		
Norco	G		
Norpace Norpace CR	G		
Norvasc	G S	felodipine, nifedipine ER	1) hydrochlorothiazide, chlorthalidone 2) atenolol, nadolol, propranolol 3) lisinopril, enalapril, captopril 4) diltiazem, verapamil 5) clonidine, guanfacine
Nuvaring		Necon	
Ogen	G S		
Omacor		USP-verified fish-oil capsules	gemfibrozil
ondansetron	S		prochlorperazine, promethazine
Oxytrol patches		oxybutinin tablets	
Pacerone	G		

*G = generic availability   **S = tablet suitable for splitting

Drug	G* S**	Same-class substitutions	Alternate-class substitutions
Parafon Forte DSC	G		
Patanol			Advanced Eye Relief, Naphcon-A, Rite Aid Eye Allergy, Visine-A
Paxil	G S		
Paxil CR		paroxetine immediate release	
Pepcid	G S		
Pexeva	G S		
Plavix	G	aspirin	dipyrimadole + aspirin
Plendil	G S		
Pletal	G S		
Ponstel		ibuprofen, naproxen	
Prandin	S		1) glipizide, glyburide, glimepiride 2) metformin
Pravachol	G S		
Pravigard		pravastatin + aspirin	
Precose	S		1) glipizide, glyburide, glimepiride 2) metformin
Prefest		[(estradiol or estropipate) + medroxyprogesterone]	
Premarin	G S	estradiol, estropipate	
Premphase		[(estradiol or estropipate) + medroxyprogesterone]	

Drug	G* S**	Same-class substitutions	Alternate-class substitutions
Prempro		[(estradiol or estropipate) + medroxyprogesterone]	
Prevacid		omeprazole	1) ranitidine, famotidine 2) OTC antacids
Prilosec	G		1) ranitidine, famotidine 2) OTC antacids
Prinivil Prinzide	G		
Procardia XL	G		
Prolixin	G		
Proscar	G		doxazosin, terazosin
Protonix		omeprazole	1) ranitidine, famotidine 2) OTC antacids
Prozac Prozac weekly	G		
Pulmicort		beclomethasone inhaler	
Relafen	G	ibuprofen, naproxen	
Relpax	S		1) aspirin, naproxen, ketoprofen 2) codeine, hydrocodone 3) prochlorperazine, promethazine 4) ergotamine tartrate 5) isometheptene/ acetaminophen 6) butalbital-APAP-caffeine
Remeron	G S		fluoxetine, paroxetine, sertraline

*G = generic availability   **S = tablet suitable for splitting

Drug	G* S**	Same-class substitutions	Alternate-class substitutions
Requip	S	For RLS: carbidopa/levodopa	For RLS: 1) propoxyphene, hydrocodone 2) clonazepam, oxazepam, zolpidem 3) gabapentin
Restoril	G S		
Rheumatrex	G		
Rhinocort Aq		flunisolide, fluticasone	1) loratidine, cetirizine 2) cromolyn sodium nasal spray
Risperdal	S		1) fluphenazine, haloperidol, thioridazine, thiothixene 2) lithium 3) carbamazepine
Ritalin	G	dexmethylphenidate, dextroamphetamine	
Ritalin LA		dextroamphetamine CR, methylphenidate	
Robaxin	G		
Rozerem		melatonin	1) zolpidem 2) lorazepam, oxazepam, temazepam
Rythmol	G S		
Sanctura		oxybutinin	amitriptyline, doxepin, nortriptyline
Sandimmune	G		
Sarafem	G	paroxetine, sertraline	
Sectral	G		

Drug	G* S**	Same-class substitutions	Alternate-class substitutions
Serevent Discus		albuterol inhaler, metaproterenol	1) beclomethasone inhaler 2) theophylline
Seroquel	S		1) fluphenazine, haloperidol, thioridazine, thiothixene 2) lithium 3) carbamazepine
Sinemet	G		
Singulair			For asthma: 1) albuterol inhaler 2) beclomethasone inhaler 3) theophylline For allergies: 1) loratidine, cetirizine 2) cromolyn sodium nasal spray
Skelaxin		orphenadrine, chlorzoxazone, cyclobenzaprine, methocarbamol	
Solodyn	G	doxycycline, tetracycline	
Soma	G	orphenadrine, chlorzoxazone, cyclobenzaprine, methocarbamol	
Sonata		zolpedem immediate release	lorazepam, oxazepam, temazepam
Sotalol	S	atenolol, metoprolol	
Spireva		atrovent inhaler, ipratropium nebulizer solution	1) albuterol inhaler 2) beclomethasone inhaler 3) theophylline

*G = generic availability   **S = tablet suitable for splitting

Drug	G* S**	Same-class substitutions	Alternate-class substitutions
Starlix	S		1) glipizide, glyburide 2) metformin
Strattera			dextroamphetamine LA, methylphenidate IR
Sular	S	felodipine, nifedipine ER	1) hydrochlorothiazide, chlorthalidone 2) atenolol, nadolol, propranolol 3) lisinopril, enalapril, captopril 4) diltiazem, verapamil 5) clonidine, guanfacine
Surmontil		amitriptyline, desipramine, doxepin, nortriptyline	
Symbicort		[(albuterol or metaproterenol inhaler) + beclomethasone inhaler]	theophylline
Symbyax			[fluoxetine + (fluphenazine, haloperidol, thioridazine, or thiothixene)]
Tambocor	G S		
Tarka		[ACE inhibitor + verapamil ER]	
Tasmar	S	entacapone	

*G = generic availability   **S = tablet suitable for splitting

Drug	G* S**	Same-class substitutions	Alternate-class substitutions
Tekturna	S		1) hydrochlorothiazide, chlorthalidone 2) atenolol, nadolol, propranolol 3) lisinopril, enalapril, captopril 4) diltiazem, verapamil, nifedipine ER 5) clonidine, guanfacine
Tenex	G S	clonidine	
Teveten/ Teveten HCT			1) hydrochlorothiazide, chlorthalidone 2) atenolol, nadolol, propranolol 3) lisinopril, enalapril, captopril 4) diltiazem, verapamil, nifedipine ER 5) clonidine, guanfacine
Thalitone	G		
Theo-24		theophylline CR tablets	
Tiazac	G	diltiazem ER	
Ticlid	G	aspirin	
Tilade			1) albuterol inhaler 2) beclomethasone inhaler 3) theophylline
Tizanidine		orphenadrine, chlorzoxazone, cyclobenzaprine, methocarbamol	
Tofranil	G S		

*G = generic availability   **S = tablet suitable for splitting

Drug	G* S**	Same-class substitutions	Alternate-class substitutions
Tolectin/ tolmetin		ibuprofen, naproxen	
Topamax	S	For migraine prevention: depakote ER	For migraine prevention: 1) atenolol, propranolol, timolol 2) desipramine, nortripyline, 3) verapamil ER
Toprol XL	G S	metoprolol immediate release	
Trandate	G S		
Transderm-Nitro		isosorbide mononitrate CR	
Tranxene-Sd	G	clorazepate immediate release, alprazolam, diazepam, lorazepam	
Travatan/ Travatan Z			1) timolol, levobunolol 2) brimonidine 3) pilocarpine
Trental	G		
Trexall	G		
Tricor		gemfibrozil	lovastatin, pravastatin, simvastatin
Trusopt			1) timolol, levobunolol 2) brimonidine 3) pilocarpine
Ultracet		tramadol + Tylenol	
Ultram/ Ultram ER	G		
Uniphyl		theophylline CR tablets	

Drug	G* S**	Same-class substitutions	Alternate-class substitutions
Uniretic	S	lisinopril/HCT, enalapril/HCT, captopril/HCT	
Univasc	S	lisinopril, enalapril, captopril	
Urispas		oxybutinin	amitriptyline, doxepin, nortriptyline
Uroxatrol		doxazosin, terazosin	
Vagifem	G	estradiol, estropipate	
Valtrex	S	acyclovir	
Vascor		diltiazem, verapamil, nifedipine ER	
Vasotec	G		
Vasoretic	G		
Venlafaxine	S		fluoxetine, paroxetine, sertraline
Veramyst	G	flunisolide, fluticasone	1) loratidine, cetirizine 2) cromolyn sodium nasal spray
Verelan/ Verelan PM	G	verapamil CR tablets	
Vesicare	S	oxybutinin	amitriptyline, doxepin, nortriptyline
Vibra-Tabs	G		
Vibramycin	G		
Vicodin/ Vicodin ES/ Vicodin HP	G		
Vicoprofen	G	hydrocodone-APAP + ibuprofen	

*G = generic availability   **S = tablet suitable for splitting

Drug	G* S**	Same-class substitutions	Alternate-class substitutions
Vistaril	G		
Vivactil		desipramine, doxepin, nortriptyline	
Vivelle/ Vivelle-Dot		estradiol, estropipate	
Voltaren XR		diclofenac immediate release, ibuprofen, naproxen	
Vytorin			lovastatin, pravastatin, simvastatin
Welchol			lovastatin, pravastatin, simvastatin
Wellbutrin/ Wellbutrin SR Wellbutrin XL	G	bupropion, bupropion 12 hour, bupropion 24 hour	fluoxetine, paroxetine, sertraline
Xalatan			1) timolol, levobunolol 2) brimonidine 3) pilocarpine
Xanax	G S		
Xanax XR		alprazolam immediate release, clonazepam	
Xopenex/ Xopenex HFA		albuterol, albuterol HFA, metaproterenol	
Xyzal		loratidine, cetirizine	cromolyn sodium nasal spray
Zaditor			Advanced Eye Relief, Naphcon-A, Rite Aid Eye Allergy, Visine-A

Drug	G* S**	Same-class substitutions	Alternate-class substitutions
Zanaflex		orphenadrine, chlorzox-azone, cyclobenzaprine, methocarbanol	
Zantac	G		
Zaroxolyn	G	hydrochlorothiazide, chlorthalidone	
Zebeta	G	atenolol, nadolol, propranolol	
Zegerid		omeprazole + bicarbonate of soda	
Zestril/ Zestoretic	G S		
Ziac	G		
Zocor	G S	lovastatin, pravastatin	
Zofran	S		prochlorperazine, promethazine
Zoloft	G S		
Zomig/ Zomig ZMT	S		1) aspirin, naproxen, ketoprofen 2) codeine, hydrocodone 3) prochlorperazine, promethazine 4) ergotamine tartrate 5) isometheptene/ acetaminophen 6) butalbital-APAP-caffeine
Zorprin		aspirin immediate release	
Zovirax	G		
Zyban	G		

*G = generic availability   **S = tablet suitable for splitting

Drug	G* S**	Same-class substitutions	Alternate-class substitutions
Zyflo			1) albuterol inhaler 2) beclomethasone inhaler 3) theophylline
Zyloprim	G		
Zyprexa	S		1) fluphenazine, haloperidol, thioridazine, thiothixene 2) lithium 3) carbamazepine

*G = generic availability   **S = tablet suitable for splitting

Endnotes

CHAPTER 1. THE TREATMENT REVIEW VISIT

1. M. Heisler et al., "Clinician identification of chronically ill patients who have problems paying for prescription medications," *American Journal of Medicine* 116 (June 1, 2004): 753–58.

2. L. S. Fields, "Medicare Part D Is Helping Seniors," *Los Angeles Times* (January 22, 2006): Business, Part C.

CHAPTER 3. ELIMINATE NONESSENTIAL PRESCRIPTIONS: COST-SAVING METHODS 1 THROUGH 4

1. A. S. Brett, "Unnecessary drug prescribing among frail elders," *Journal Watch* 25 (November 1, 2005): 167.

2. E. R. Hajjar et al., "Unnecessary drug use in frail older people at hospital discharge," *Journal of the American Geriatric Society* 53 (September 2005): 1518–23.

3. C. Zhan, J. Sandl, A. S. Biermand, et al., "Potentially inappropriate medication use in the community-dwelling elderly. Findings from the 1996 Medical Expenditure Panel Survey," *Journal of the American Medical Association* 286, 22 (December 2001): 2823–29.

4. M. Salas et al. "Are proton pump inhibitors the first choice for acute treatment of gastric ulcers? A meta analysis of randomized clinical trials," *BMC Gastroenterology* 2 (2002): 17.

5. Y. Yang et al., "Long-term proton pump inhibitor therapy and risk of hip fracture," *Journal of the American Medical Association* 296 (2006): 2947–53.

6. American Psychiatric Association, *Practice Guideline for the Treatment of Patients with Major Depressive Disorder*, 2nd ed. (Washington, D.C.: American Psychiatric Association, 2000).

7. C. F. Reynolds et al., "Maintenance treatment of major depression in old age," *New England Journal of Medicine* 354 (March 16, 2006): 1189–90.

8. H. G. Bone et al., "Ten years' experience with alendronate for osteo-
    porosis in post-menopausal women," *New England Journal of Medicine*
    350 (2004): 1189; D. M. Black et al., "Effects of continuing or stopping
    alendronate after five years treatment," *Journal of the American Medi-
    cal Association* 296 (2006): 2927–38.

9. C. V. Odvina et al., "Severely suppressed bone turnover: A potential
    complication of alendronate therapy," *Journal of Clinical Endocrinol-
    ogy and Metabolism* 90 (March 2005): 1294–1301.

10. S. E. Kahn et al., "Glycemic durability of rosiglitazone, metformin,
    or glyburide monotherapy," *New England Journal of Medicine* 355
    (December 2006): 2427–43.

11. AD2000 Collaborative Group, "Long-term donazepril treatment
    in 565 patients with Alzheimer's disease (AD2000): Randomized
    double-blind trial," *Lancet* 363 (June 26, 2004): 2105–15.

12. B. M. Kuehm, "FDA warns antipsychotic drugs may be risky for
    elderly," *Journal of the American Medical Association* 293 (2005):
    2462.

13. K. M. Sink et al., "Pharmacological treatment of neuropsychiatric
    symptoms of dementia: A review of the evidence," *Journal of the
    American Medical Association* 293 (2005): 596.

14. H. S. Nelson, et al., "The salmeterol multicenter asthma research
    trial: A comparison of usual pharmacotherapy for asthma or usual
    pharmacotherapy plus salmeterol," *Chest* 129 (January 2006):
    15–26.

15. www.fda.gov/Cder/drug/InfoSheets/HCP/fluticasoneHCP.htm

16. T. G. Pickering, "Ambulatory blood pressure monitoring in clinical
    practice," *Clinical Cardiology* 14 (1991): 557–62.

CHAPTER 4. THINKING OUTSIDE THE PRESCRIPTION DRUG BOTTLE: COST-SAVING METHODS 5 THROUGH 7

1. E. A. McGlynn, S. M. Asch, J. Adams, et al., "The quality of health
    care delivered to adults in the United States," *New England Journal
    of Medicine* 348 (2003): 2635–45.

2. National Heart, Lung, and Blood Institute, "The Seventh Report of Joint National Committee on Prevention, Detection, Evaluation, and Treatment of High Blood Pressure," NIH Publication no. 04–5230, August 2004.

3. JNC 7 Express, "The Seventh Report of Joint National Committee on Prevention, Detection, Evaluation, and Treatment of High Blood Pressure" NIH Publication no. 03–5233, December 2003.

4. R. J. Barnard, S. C. DiLauro, and S. B. Inkeles, "Effects of intensive diet and exercise intervention in patients taking cholesterol-lowering drugs," *American Journal of Cardiology* 79, no. 8 (April 15, 1997): 1112–14.

5. J. Lexchin, "Pharmaceutical industry sponsorship and research outcome and quality: systematic review," *British Medical Journal* 326 (May 29, 2003): 1167–70, www.bmj.com/cgi/content/full/326/7400/1167.

6. J. A. Cauley, J. Robbins, et al., "Effects of estrogen plus progestin on risk of fracture and bone mineral density: The Women's Health Initiative randomized trial," *Journal of the American Medical Association* 290 (2003): 1729–38; Women's Health Initiative Steering Committee, "Effects of conjugated equine estrogen in postmenopausal women with hysterectomy: The Women's Health Initiative randomized controlled trial," *Journal of the American Medical Association* 291 (2004): 1701–12; S. Wassertheil-Smoller, S. Hendrix, M. Limacher, "Effect of estrogen plus progestin on stroke in postmenopausal women: The Women's Health Initiative: A randomized trial," *Journal of the American Medical Association* 289 (2003): 2673–84.

7. J. E. Rossouw et al., "Risks and benefits of estrogen plus progestin in healthy postmenopausal women: Principal results from the Women's Health Initiative randomized controlled trial," *Journal of the American Medical Association* 288 (2002): 321–33.

8. A. Radtke et al., "Self treatment of benign paroxysmal positional vertigo: Semont maneuver vs Epley procedure," *Neurology* 63 (July 13, 2004): 150–52.

9. K. J. Sherman et al., "Comparing yoga, exercise, and a self-care book for chronic low back pain: A randomized, controlled trial," *Annals of Internal Medicine* 143 (December 20, 2005): 849–56.

10. A. J. Lang, "Treating generalized anxiety disorder with cognitive-behavioral therapy," *Journal of Clinical Psychiatry* 65, Suppl., no. 13 (2004): 14; M.W. Otto et al., "Cognitive-behavioral therapy for the treatment of anxiety disorders," *Journal of Clinical Psychiatry* 65, Suppl., no. 5 (2004): 34.

11. C. E. D. H. De Laet et al., "Bone density and risk of hip fracture in men and women: Cross-sectional analysis," *British Medical Journal* 325 (1997): 221–25.

12. www.imshealth.com/ims/portal/front/articleC/ 0,2777,6599_77685 579_77685588,00.html

13. P. W. F. Wilson et al., "Prediction of coronary heart disease using risk factor categories," *Circulation* 97 (1998): 1837–47.

14. J. Shepherd, S. M. Cobb, I. Ford, et al. "Prevention of coronary heart disease with pravastatin in men with hypercholesterolemia," *New England Journal of Medicine* 333 (1995): 1301–07.

15. P. S. Sever, B. Dahlof, N. R. Poulter, et al., "Prevention of coronary and stroke events with atorvastatin in hypertensive patients who have average or lower-than-average cholesterol concentrations in the Anglo-Scandinavian cardiac outcomes trial—lipid-lowering arm (ASCOT-LLA): A multicenter randomized controlled trial," *Lancet* 361 (2003): 1149–58; J. R. Downs, M. Clearfield, S. Weis, et al., "Primary prevention of acute coronary events with lovastatin in men and women with average cholesterol levels: Results of AFCAPS/TexCAPS," *Journal of the American Medical Association* 279 (1998): 1615–22.

16. J. Shepherd, G. J. Blauw, M. B. Murphy, et al., "Pravastatin in elderly individuals at risk of vascular disease (PROSPER): A randomized controlled trial," *Lancet* http://image.thelancet.com/extras/02art8325web.pdf

17. B. M. Psaty et al., "The association between lipid levels and the risks of incident myocardial infarction, stroke, and total mortality:

The cardiovascular study," *Journal of the American Geriatric Society* 52 (October 2004): 1639–47.

18. S. N. Blair, H. W. Kohl, C. E. Barlow, et al. "Changes in physical fitness and all-cause mortality: A prospective study of healthy and unhealthy men," *Journal of the American Medical Association* 273 (1995): 1093–98.

19. S. E. Sherman et al., "Does exercise reduce mortality rates in the elderly? Experience from the Framingham heart study," *American Heart Journal* 128, no. 5 (November 1994): 965–72.

20. I. S. Ockene and N. H. Miller, "Cigarette smoking, cardiovascular disease, and stroke," *Circulation* 96 (1997): 3243–47.

21. A. Trichopoulou et al., "Modified Mediterranean diet and survival: EPIC-elderly prospective cohort study," *British Medical Journal* 5: 271–75.

22. M. de Lorgeril, P. Salen, J. L. Martin, et al., "Mediterranean diet, traditional risk factors, and the rate of cardiovascular complications after myocardial infarction: Final report of the Lyon diet heart study," *Circulation* 99, no. 6 (1999): 779–85; P. Kris-Etherton, R. H. Eckel, B. V. Howard, et al., "AHA science advisory. Lyon diet heart study: Benefits of a Mediterranean-style, national cholesterol education program/American Heart Association step I dietary pattern on cardiovascular disease," Circulation 103, no. 13 (2001): 1823–25.

23. S. Yusef et al., "Effect of potentially modifiable risk factors associated with myocardial infarction in 52 countries (the INTERHEART study): Case-control study," *Lancet* 364 (September 11, 2004): 937–52.

24. J. M. Froody et al., "Hydroxymethylglutaryl-CoA reductase inhibitors in older persons with acute myocardial infarction: Evidence for an age statin interaction," *Journal of the American Geriatric Society* 54 (March 2006): 421–30.

25. R. A. Hayward et al., "Narrative review: Lack of evidence for recommended low-density lipoprotein treatment targets: A solvable problem," *Annals of Internal Medicine* 145 (October 3, 2006): 520–30.

26. C. Patrono et al., "Low-dose aspirin for the prevention of atherthombosis," *New England Journal of Medicine* 353 (2005): 2373–83; J. S. Berger et al., "Aspirin for the primary prevention of cardiovascular events in women and men: A sex-specific meta-analysis of randomized controlled trials," *Journal of the American Medical Association* 295 (2006): 306.

27. World Health Organization Collaborating Centre for Metabolic Bone Diseases, "FAQ," *FRAX: WHO Fracture Risk Assessment Tool*, University of Sheffield, UK. http://www.shef.ac.uk/FRAX/faq.htm

28. S. R. Cummings et al., "Effect of alendronate on risk of fracture in women with low bone density but without vertebral fractures," *Journal of the American Medical Association* 280 (December 1998): 2077–82.

29. M. R. McClung, P. Geusens, P. D. Miller, et al., "Effect of residronate on the risk of hip fracture in elderly women," *New England Journal of Medicine* 344, no. 5 (2001): 333–40.

30. C. H. Chestnut III et al., "Effects of oral ibandronate administered daily or intermittently on fracture risk in postmenopausal osteoporosis," *Journal of Bone and Mineral Research* 19 (2004): 1241.

31. E. W. Gregg et al., "Physical activity and osteoporotic fracture risk in older women," *Annals of Internal Medicine* 129 (July 15, 1998): 81–88; D. Feskanich, et al., "Walking and leisure-time activity and risk of hip fracture in postmenopausal women," *Journal of the American Medical Association* 288 (November 13, 2002): 2300–2306.

32. H. A. Bischoff-Ferrari et al., "Fracture prevention with vitamin D supplementation: A meta-analysis of randomized controlled trials," *Journal of the American Medical Association* 293 (May 11, 2005): 2257–64; D. P. Trivedi et al., "Effect of four monthly oral vitamin D_3 (cholecalciferol) supplementation on fractures and mortality in men and women living in the community: Randomized double blind controlled trial," *British Medical Journal* 326 (March 1, 2003): 469–72; M. C. Chapuy et al., "Vitamin D3 and calcium to prevent

hip fractures in elderly women," *New England Journal of Medicine* 327 (December 3, 1992): 1637–42.

33. Y. Sato et al., "Effect of folate and mecobalamin on hip fractures in patients with stroke: A randomized controlled trial," *Journal of the American Medical Association* 293 (March 2, 2005): 1082–88.

34. L. A. Frassetto, "Worldwide incidence of hip fracture in elderly women: relation to consumption of animal and vegetable foods," *Journals of Gerontology Series A: Biological Sciences and Medical Sciences* 55, no. 10 (October 2000): M585–92.

35. P. Kannus et al., "Prevention of hip fracture in elderly people with use of a hip protector," *New England Journal of Medicine* 343 (November 2000): 1506–13; J. B. Lauritzen, M. M. Petersen, and B. Lund. "Effect of external hip protectors on hip fractures," *Lancet* 341 (1993): 11–13; M. J. Parker, L. D. Gillespie, and W. J. Gillespie. "Hip protectors for preventing hip fractures in the elderly [review]," *Cochrane Database of Systematic Reviews* 2 (2001): CD001255.

36. J. Jensen, "Fall and injury prevention in older people living in residential care facilities:, A cluster randomized trial," *Annals of Internal Medicine* 136 (2002): 733–41.

37. National Osteoporosis Foundation, Clinician's Guide to Prevention and Treatment of Osteoporosis, www.nof.org/professionals/ NOF_Clincians_Guide.pdf

CHAPTER 5. STEER CLEAR OF OVERPRICED REDUNDANT DRUGS: COST-SAVING METHODS 8 THROUGH 12

1. S. G. Morgan et al., "'Breakthrough' drugs and growth in expenditure on prescription drugs in Canada," *British Medical Journal* 5 (2005): 511–12.

2. M. Angell. *The Truth about the Drug Companies.* (New York: Random House, 2004).

3. Canadian Institute for Health Information. *Drug Expenditures in Canada 1985–2004* (Ottawa: CIHI, 2005).

4. Federal Food, Drug, and Cosmetic (FD&C) Act, Title 21, Code of Federal Regulations [CFR] section 202.1. View the guidance at www.fda.gov/cder/guidance/1804fnl.htm

5. R. Frank et al., "Trends in direct-to-consumer advertising of prescription drugs" Kaiser Family Foundation, February 2002.

6. Advertising Educational Foundation, "Ten years later: direct to consumer drug advertising," www.aef.com/industry/news/data/2006/6084.

7. R. L. Kravitz et al., "Influence of patients' requests for direct-to-consumer advertised antidepressants: A randomized controlled trial," *Journal of the American Medical Association* 293 (April 27, 2005): 1995–2002.

8. *The Medical Letter on Drugs and Therapeutics* 46, no. 1189 (August 2004): 65.

9. "FDA oversight of direct-to-consumer advertising has limitations," www.gao.gov/new.items/d03177.pdf.

10. G. D. Curfman et al., "Expression of concern: Bombardier et al., comparison of upper gastrointestinal toxicity of rofecoxib and naprosyn in patients with rhuematoid arthritis," *New England Journal of Medicine* 343 (2000): 1520–28, 353 (2005): 2813–14.

11. U.S. Food and Drug Administration, "Safety-based drug withdrawals (1997–2001)," *FDA Consumer* 36, no. 1 (January–February 2002) www.fda.gov/fdac/features/2002/chrtWithdrawls.html.

12. B. M. Psaty et al., "Potential for conflict of interest in the evaluation of suspected adverse drug reactions: Use of cerivastatin and risk of rhabdomyolosis," *Journal of the American Medical Association* 292 (December 2004): 2622–31.

13. D. J. Grahm et al., "Incidence of hospitalized rhabdomyolosis in patients treated with lipid-lowering drugs," *Journal of the American Medical Association* 292 (December 2004): 2585–90.

14. Law offices of Dana Taschner, "Rezulin linked to liver failure and heart disease," *Drug Recalls* www.drugrecalls.com/rezulin.html.

15. S. D. Solomon et al., "Cardiovascular risk associated with celecoxib in a clinical trial for colorectal adenoma prevention," *New England Journal of Medicine* 352 (March 2005): 1071–80.

16. B. Soloway and A. S. Brett, "More data on COX-2 inhibitors," *Journal Watch* 25 (March 15, 2005): 45–46.

17. "Generic drugs." *The Medical Letter on Drugs and Therapeutics* 44 (2002): 89.

18. A. Smith, "FDA backlog = billions for big pharma?" *CNNMoney.com* (April 10, 2006), http://money.cnn.com/2006/04/10/news/companies /fdabacklog/index.htm.

19. B. M. Psaty et al., "The risk of myocardial infarction associated with antihypertensive drug therapies," *Journal of the American Medical Association* 274, no. 8 (August 23, 1995): 620–25.

20. S. Yusuf et al., "Effects of an angiotensin-converting–enzyme inhibitor, Ramipril, on cardiovascular events in high-risk patients," *New England Journal of Medicine* 342 (2000): 145–52.

21. L. Pilote, "Mortality rates in elderly patients who take different angiotensin-converting enzyme inhibitors after acute myocardial infarction: A class effect?" *Annals of Internal Medicine* 141 (July 20, 2004): 102–112.

22. F. M. Sacks, "High-intensity statin treatment for coronary disease" *Journal of the American Medical Association* 291 (March 3, 2004): 1132–34.

23. T. R. Pedersen et al., "High-dose atorvastatin versus usual-dose simvistatin for secondary prevention after myocardial infarction, The IDEAL study: A randomized controlled trial," *Journal of American Medical Association* 294 (November 16, 2005): 2437–45.

24. *Medical Letter on Drugs and Therapeutics* 45 (2003): 93–95.

25. G. Schernthaner et al. "Efficacy and safety of pioglitazone versus metformin in patients with type II diabetes mellitus: A double-blind randomized trial," *Journal of Clinical Endocrinol and Metabolism* 89 (December 2004): 6068–76.

26. S. Singh et al., "Long-term risk of cardiovascular events with Rosigli-tazone," *Journal of the American Medical Association* 298, no. 10 (2007): 1189–95.

27. I. Raz et al., "Efficacy and safety of the dipeptidyl peptidase-4 inhibi-tor sitagliptin as monotherapy in patients with type 2 diabetes mel-litus," *Diabetologia* 49 (2006): 2564; P. Aschner et al., "Effect of the dipeptidyl peptidase-4 inhibitor sitagliptin as monotherapy on glyce-mic control in patients with type 2 diabetes," *Diabetes Care* 29 (2006): 2632; D. M. Natan et al., "Management of hyperglycemia in type 2 diabetes: A consensus algorithm for the initiation and adjustment of therapy," *Diabetes Care* 29 (2006): 2638.

28. JNC 7 Express, "The Seventh Report of Joint National Committee on Prevention, Detection, Evaluation, and Treatment of High Blood Pressure" NIH Publication no. 03–5233, December 2003.

CHAPTER 6: PLAY IT SMART: COST-SAVING METHODS 13 THROUGH 17

1. J. E. Polli, S. Kim, and B. R. Martin. "Weight uniformity of split tablets required by a Veterans Affairs policy," *Journal of Managed Care Pharmacy* 9, no. 5 (September-October 2003): 401–407.

2. J. M. Rosenberg et al., "Weight variability of pharmacist-dispensed split tablets," *Journal of the American Pharmacists Association* 42 (2002): 200; J. Teng, et al., "Lack of medication dose uniformity in com-monly split tablets," *Journal of the American Pharmacists Association* 42 (2002): 195.

3. M. C. Duncan et al., "Effect of tablet splitting on serum choles-terol concentrations," *Annals of Pharmacotherapy* 36 (2002): 205; M. Gee et al., "Effects of a tablet-splitting program in patients taking H MG-CoA reductase inhibitors: Analysis of clinical effects, patient satisfaction, compliance, and cost avoidance," *Journal of Managed Care Pharmacy* 6 (2002): 453.

4. J. P. Rindone, "Evaluation of tablet-splitting in patients taking lisino-pril for hypertension," *Journal of Clinical Outcomes Management* 7 (2000): 22.

5. *Medical Letter on Drugs and Therapeutics*, 48, no. 1237 (June 19, 2006).

6. E. Bruckert, P. Giral, H. M. Heshmati, and G. Turpin, "Men treated with hypolipidaemic drugs complain more frequently of erectile dysfunction," *Journal of Clinical Pharmacology and Therapeutics* 21 (1996): 89–94.

7. *Medical Letter on Drugs and Therapeutics* 46, no. 1196 (November 22, 2004).

8. M. A. Omar and J. P. Wilson. "FDA adverse event reports on statin-associated rhabdomyolysis," *Annals of Pharmacotherapy* 36 (2002): 288–95.

9. S. Shrivastava, M. S. Kochar, "The dual risks of depression and hypertension," *Postgraduate Medicine Online* (June 2002) www.postgradmed.com/issues/2002/06_02/shrivastava.htm

10. T. A. Brennan et al., "Health industry practices that create conflicts of interest," *Journal of the American Medical Association* 295 (January 2006): 429–33.

11. "Impact of direct-to-consumer advertising on prescription drug spending," The Henry J. Kaiser Family Foundation. June 2003.

CHAPTER 7: PROGRAMS FOR PILLS: COST-SAVING METHODS 18 THROUGH 20

1. "GlaxoSmithKline offers new tools to help patients get free medicines," press release (February 13, 2007) www.bridgestoaccess.com/pdfs/PressRelease20070414b.pdf.

2. "Merck launches new consumer health resource, *Guide to Affordable Medicine*," press release (February 7, 2007) www.merck.com/newsroom/press_releases/corporate/2006_0207.html.

3. "Living our values," *Abbott 2004 Global Citizenship Report* (August 2005) www.abbott.com/en_US/content/document/2004gcr.pdf

4. "Fact sheet: How the pharmaceutical industry helps America's Uninsured" www.pparx.org/help_uninsured.php.

5. www.consumeraffairs.com/news04/pbms.html

6. J. Hoadley, E. Hargrave, J. Cubanski, et al, "Medicare part D 2008 data spotlight: Premiums," Kaiser Family Foundation, November 2007.

7. Juliette Cubanski, Tricia Neuman, "Overview of Medicare part D organizations, plans, and benefits by enrollment in 2006 and 2007" Kaiser Family Foundation. November 2007.

8. According to the Centers for Medicare and Medicaid Services.

9. J. Hoadley, E. Hargrave, J. Cubanski, et al., "Medicare part D 2008 data spotlight: Benefit design," Kaiser Family Foundation. December 2007.

10. J. Hoadley, E. Hargrave, J. Cubanski, et al, "Medicare part D 2008 data spotlight: The coverage gap," Kaiser Family Foundation. November 2007.

A NOTE ON EXPIRATION DATES

1. "Revision of product dating specifications," *American Journal of Health-System Pharmacy* 57 (2000): 1441–45. www.medscape.com/viewarticle/406903_2

2. *Medical Letter on Drugs and Therapeutics* 44, no. W1142B (October 28, 2002).

3. J. S. Taylor et al., "Stability profiles of drug products extended beyond labeled expiration dates," 2002 FDA science forum poster abstract, Board AC-08, www.cfsan.fda.gov/~frf/forum02/abs02ct.html#sz

4. G. Stark et al., *Pharmaceutical Journal* 258 (1997): 637.

5. C. Scholtissek and R. G. Webster, *Antiviral Research* 38 (1998): 213.

6. R. Regenthal et al., *Human and Experimental Toxicology* 21 (2002): 343.

7. G. W. Frimpter et al., *Journal of the American Medical Association* 184 (1963): 111.

8. *Medical Letter on Drugs and Therapeutics* 44, no. W1142B (October 28, 2002).

General Index